Critical Care Focus

3: Neurological Injury

EDITOR

DR HELEN F GALLEY

Lecturer in Anaesthesia and Intensive Care
University of Aberdeen

EDITORIAL BOARD

PROFESSOR NIGEL R WEBSTER

Professor of Anaesthesia and Intensive Care
University of Aberdeen

DR PAUL G P LAWLER

Clinical Director of Intensive Care
South Cleveland Hospital

DR NEIL SONI

Consultant in Anaesthesia and Intensive Care
Chelsea and Westminster Hospital

DR MERVYN SINGER

Reader in Intensive Care
University College Hospital, London

BMJ
Books

© BMJ Books 2000

BMJ Books is an imprint of the BMJ Publishing Group

First published in 2000
Second Impression 2000
Third Impression 2001

by BMJ Books, BMA House, Tavistock Square,
London WC1H 9JR

www.bmjbooks.com

British Library Cataloguing in Publication Data

A catalogue record for this book is available from the British Library

ISBN 0-7279-1596-7

Typeset by Phoenix Photosetting, Chatham, Kent
Printed and bound by Selwood Printing Ltd. West Sussex

Contents

Contributors

Peter JD Andrews
Consultant in Anaesthesia and Intensive Care, Western General Hospital, Edinburgh, UK

Daniele C Bryden
Consultant Anaesthetist, Hope Hospital, Salford, UK

Roger E Cull
Consultant Clinical Neurophysiologist, Western General Hospital, Edinburgh, UK

I Robert Ghosh
Senior Registrar, Departments of General Medicine, Intensive Care Medicine and Clinical Neurophysiology, St Bartholomew's Hospital and The London NHS Trust, London, UK

Neil R Grubb
Clinical Lecturer, University of Edinburgh Cardiovascular Unit, UK

Graham R Nimmo
Consultant Physician, Royal Infirmary of Edinburgh and Consultant Acute Physician, Western General Hospital, Edinburgh, UK

Michael G O'Sullivan
Consultant Neurosurgeon, Western General Hospital, Edinburgh, UK

Introduction

This is the third in the series of the 'State of the Art' volumes focusing on key issues in Critical Care Medicine. The series is taken from transcriptions of lectures given at Intensive Care Society meetings by renowned international experts. This third book concentrates on issues related to neurological injury and includes chapters on aspects of medical and surgical management of patients after sub-arachnoid haemorrhage, neurological injury after cardiac arrest and the role of goal oriented therapy for head injury.

Goal directed therapy for managing head injury
Daniele C Bryden

Mortality from head injury has declined markedly over the past 20 years due to improvements in monitoring underlying pathophysiological processess, imaging modalities and monitoring techniques for the injured brain. Over the last 5–10 years, there has been a fundamental change in the way in which adults with a closed head injury are managed on the intensive care unit. The emphasis has moved from primarily control of intracranial pressure to a more multifaceted approach, in particular, attention to the maintenance of cerebral perfusion pressure. This review describes the background behind one of the major current strategies for severe head injury management and assesses the implications for future practice.

Severe brain insult in the intensive care unit: neurophysiological and clinical assessment of outcome
I Robert Ghosh

The prediction of outcome after brain insult is a common challenge to all clinicians. Increasing numbers of patients are surviving the initial critical event as a direct consequence of improved facilities for immediate resuscitation in the emergency room and intensive care unit. The cessation of treatment in the setting of potentially reversible brain dysfunction is disastrous, while continuing therapy in the face of inevitable brain death is both inhumane and costly. Novel methods of assessment which provide timely reliable identification of a clear optimistic or pessimistic outlook should be encouraged. This review addresses the problems associated with the clinical and neurophysiological determination of outcome in patients with severe brain injury.

Surgical and radiological treatment of sub-arachnoid haemorrhage
Michael G O'Sullivan

During the last three decades, new diagnostic techniques and therapeutic strategies have emerged for patients with sub-arachnoid haemorrhage. The introduction of CT and catheter angiography has improved the accuracy of diagnosis and provided a tool in the evaluation of the clinical course. The application of the operating microscope has refined microsurgical techniques. More recently, the calcium antagonist nimodipine has been shown to improve outcome. Since fluid restriction and the use of antihypertensive drugs were found to be harmful, hypervolaemia, haemodilution, and in some instances even induced hypertension have been advocated. Moreover, the timing of surgery has shifted for certain categories of patients from late (>10 days) to early (0–3 days) after the initial haemorrhage. Delayed cerebral ischaemia is the major cause of death and disability in patients who initially susrvive an aneurysmal sub-arachnoid haemorrhage.

Medical management of complications following aneurysmal sub-arachnoid haemorrhage
Peter JD Andrews

This review addresses the medical management of patients who are admitted to the intensive care unit with complications following aneurysmal sub-arachnoid haemorrhage. It focuses primarily on cardiac, pulmonary and metabolic complications, and also delayed neurological deficit. It is still not entirely clear whether delayed neurological deficit is due to a failure of oxygen delivery caused by narrowing of the cerebral arterial vessels as has been assumed. Clinically there is an increase in transcranial Doppler velocities, angiographic arterial vessel narrowing and a reduction in consciousness. Recent research has also demonstrated that it is possible to monitor impending neurological deficit in the intensive care unit setting and this is discussed.

Sub-arachnoid haemorrhage: case presentation
Graham R Nimmo

The remit of this chapter is to present an example of a case of aneurysmal sub-arachnoid haemorrhage and try to highlight some of the problems in the management of this type of patient.

Sub-clinical seizures in the critically ill

Roger E Cull

This chapter provides a basic understanding of the types of seizures which may present on the intensive care unit. Neurophysiologists are quite often asked the question "Is this patient unconscious because they are having sub-clinical seizures?" and in my experience a positive answer is relatively unusual. Compared with other causes of unconsciousness in ITU patients, sub-clinical epileptic seizures are relatively uncommon.

Neurological injury in out-of-hospital cardiac arrest survivors: implications for management

Neil R Grubb and Graham R Nimmo

There is now an increasing population of cardiac arrest victims who survive with lethal or non-lethal brain injury. Of those who survive and are admitted to hospital, at least a third require management in an intensive care unit, mainly because of failure to spontaneously ventilate and self-oxygenate. These resuscitated cardiac arrest victims present a challenge to intensivists in terms of assessing and managing neurological injury.

1: Goal directed therapy for managing head injury

DANIELE C BRYDEN

Introduction

Mortality from head injury has declined markedly over the past twenty years. Advances have occurred in our knowledge of the underlying pathophysiological processes, imaging modalities and monitoring techniques for the injured brain.[1] General intensive care practice has also improved, such that it is very difficult to identify the relative contributions to improvement in survival. Furthermore, current UK practice varies widely both within neurosurgical and non-specialist intensive care centres, in terms of the availability of patient monitoring and the treatments utilised. It is difficult therefore to carry out any multicentre studies or comparison of units.[2,3]

It is clear that over the past 5–10 years, there has been a fundamental change in the way in which adults with a closed head injury are managed on the intensive care unit (ICU). The emphasis has moved from primarily control of intracranial pressure (ICP) to a more multifaceted approach; in particular, attention to the maintenance of cerebral perfusion pressure (CPP). This review describes the background behind one of the major current strategies for severe head injury management (Glasgow Coma Score (GCS) ≤ 8) and assesses the implications for future practice.

The scope of the problem

Real progress has been made in the treatment of the injured brain, yet adult head injuries are responsible for 70% of accidental deaths and persisting disability after trauma. Many victims are young, which places a significant social and financial strain on their families when the outcome is poor.[4] Improvements in the quality of anaesthesia for neurosurgery have facilitated surgical progress, minimising brain insult at the time of operation, and the value of optimal intensive care management for patients with severe head injury is widely accepted. Why then, given the clear improvements in the quality of surgery, anaesthesia, and intensive care, does head injury continue to be so devastating? Current literature suggests that although there is great variation in the types of pathological processes that occur in relation to the primary injury, there is even greater disagreement in the way in which the injured brain should subsequently be treated.[5-7]

Physiological principles

The importance of maintaining adequate cerebral oxygen delivery is not disputed, and can be achieved by maintaining adequate circulating volume, oxygenation, and perfusion pressures.[8] The brain does not differ from any other injured organ in this respect, but is disadvantaged by being encased within the rigid confines of the skull. Imaging and monitoring are therefore more difficult, and there is a greater susceptibility to swelling from oedema formation. Under normal circumstances the brain is able to regulate its own blood flow, such that supply of oxygen and substrate is always sufficient to meet metabolic demand. Cerebral autoregulation maintains blood flow over a wide range of cerebral perfusion pressures. Healthy individuals are able to maintain adequate cerebral blood flow over a wide range of mean arterial blood pressures, so that in the absence of intracranial hypertension, blood flow within the brain is essentially independent of perfusion pressure. Perhaps even more important is the fact that any initial injury can be exacerbated by other undesirable and often preventable physiological insults, leading to secondary neurological injury and further deterioration. Inattention to preventing secondary injury in the early resuscitation phase will make subsequent intensive care management more problematical and worsen the overall outcome.[9]

Conventional approaches to head injury: control of intracranial pressure

In the past control of intracranial pressure was regarded as the mainstay in preventing the secondary insults that can ultimately lead to cerebral herniation and death.[10,11] The traditional approach was based on therapy to reduce the cerebral oedema formed as a natural sequel to the injury.[4] This can be achieved by hyperventilation, control of fluid balance, avoidance of hypertension, and, wherever possible, maintenance of ICP below a predetermined level. This strategy evolved from the supposition that after a head injury, paralysis of the cerebral vasculature occurs, resulting in

2

widespread cerebral vasodilatation. Cerebral blood flow subsequently appeared to become entirely dependent on perfusion pressure, so that at higher perfusion pressures, a large component of the rise in ICP was thought to be due to hyperaemia. This concept was first proposed over 30 years ago to explain the cerebral oedema and intracranial hypertension seen after experimental studies of head injury.[12,13] This naturally led to the assumption that strict control of blood pressure was necessary to limit the hyperaemic contribution of cerebral blood flow to the rise in intracranial pressure. In addition to hyperaemic and ischaemic causes of secondary neuronal injury, the development of vasogenic tissue oedema could be prevented by avoidance of overhydration and surges in blood pressure.

It has never been shown definitively that lowering ICP in patients with intracranial hypertension improves outcome from severe traumatic brain injury.[10,14] However, an ICP of greater than 20 mmHg has been shown by Marmarou *et al.* to be the fourth most powerful predictor of outcome after age, admission GCS, and pupillary signs.[11] Management strategies aimed at controlling ICP have therefore always been attractive. Unfortunately, the confounding effects on CPP of reducing ICP and compromising cerebral blood flow were often not considered and therefore inadequately controlled. Although half the deaths from head injury are caused by uncontrolled ICP, it has been suggested that considerable morbidity may result from attempts to control ICP at a predetermined level. Unfortunately ethical considerations may preclude a definitive study, although evidence suggests that treatment for intracranial hypertension should be initiated at 20–25 mmHg.[10] In addition, therapies aimed at controlling ICP may have an inherent associated morbidity without, as in the case of hyperventilation, any evidence of benefit when give empirically.[15] Although evidence for the importance of an adequate CPP does not come from randomised controlled trials, a correlation between mortality and CPP has been shown.[16] Many severe head injury patients require a cerebral perfusion pressure of 60–70 mmHg to reduce ischaemic insults, although the actual level can vary greatly between individuals.[17] It is possible that therapies aimed at maintaining CPP, rather than lowering ICP, may be a more rational therapeutic goal.[18]

Control of cerebral perfusion pressure

The premise for maintenance of CPP is the manipulation of autoregulatory responses in an intact but potentially abnormal cerebral vasculature (Figure 1.1). This has been suggested in part from the observation of the cyclical rises in ICP in response to falls in blood pressure (and therefore CPP) first described in 1928 by Wolff and Forbes[19] and later by Lundberg.[20] Plateau or A waves are spontaneous acute rises in ICP

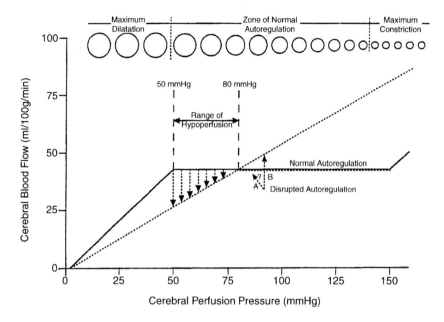

Figure 1.1 Schematic diagram demonstrating the relationship between cerebral blood vessel diameter, cerebral perfusion pressure, and cerebral blood flow. Reproduced with permission from Narayan RK. Neurotrauma. New York: McGraw-Hill, 1996.

above a slightly elevated baseline pressure and can last up to 30 minutes, with ICP usually returning to baseline levels fairly rapidly. *In vitro* and *in vivo* animal studies have demonstrated that plateau waves are a direct result of falls in CPP, and may reflect the attempts of an intact cerebral autoregulatory system to maintain an adequate cerebral blood flow by means of increasing vessel diameter.[21] The cerebral vasodilatation that occurs during these rises in ICP always reduces CPP if blood pressure is unchanged, and may even ultimately compromise cerebral blood flow. This is not surprising given the mathematical relationship between ICP and CPP. Rapid restoration of CPP may result in termination of the rise in ICP, with a so-called "termination spike" in ICP prior to the subsequent decrease (Figure 1.2). This termination spike was described initially by Cushing, when rises in blood pressure were seen in response to ischaemia of the vasomotor centre as an attempt to maintain the cerebral circulation in the face of intracranial hypertension.[22,23]

It can therefore be inferred that control of CPP (and blood pressure) will help to prevent any additional ischaemia and the development of intracranial pressure waves. The observed pressure wave formation may be described in terms of cascades of cerebral blood vessel vasoconstriction and vasodilatation (Figure 1.3).

4

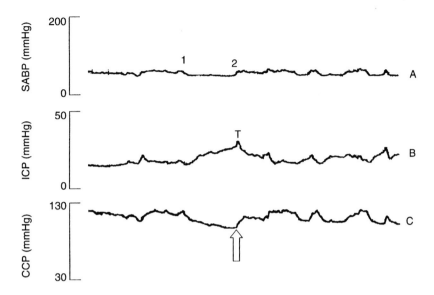

*Figure 1.2   The clinical relationship between intracranial pressure (ICP) and cerebral perfusion pressure (CPP). **A** Reduction in CPP stimulated by spontaneous 15 mmHg decrease in systemic arterial blood pressure (SABP) (1). ICP increased and further lowered CPP because SABP did not change; this continued until CPP increased as a result of SABP reaching 100 mmHg (2). The progress of (1) to (2) demonstrates a self-sustaining vasodilatory cascade. **B** The initial passive increase in ICP (T = termination spike) before ICP decreased. **C** The "ischaemic threshold" is between 60 and 70 mmHg (arrow), useful in selecting a minimum CPP (in this case above 70 mmHg). However, lowest ICP occurs at CPP of 85–90 mmHg, which is better as an optimal target CPP, rather than the minimal value. The relationships change as brain injury evolves and both higher and lower optimal CPP values can be identified. Reproduced with permission from Rosner MJ et al. J Neurosurg 1995;**83**:949–62.[18]*

The vasoconstriction–vasodilatation cascade

Vasoreactivity is brought about in response to changes in CPP by alterations in the vascular tone of the cerebral arterioles, although the range over which this occurs is limited. In normal circumstances, at the upper inflexion point of the autoregulation curve, cerebral vessels are maximally constricted, but at lower perfusion pressures, they dilate in an attempt to maintain cerebral blood flow. Vessel diameter does not change in a linear fashion, but alters logarithmically, with maximal changes occurring in the range of CPP values between 50 and 80 mmHg.[24] Below the lower autoregulation limit, changes in vessel diameter are passive, and vessels begin to collapse in response to the falling perfusion pressure, their diameter being determined primarily by transmural pressure. This is demonstrated schematically in Figure 1.1. The net result is a severe impairment in cerebral blood flow, with ischaemia if cerebral metabolism remains unchanged.

Vasodilatory cascade

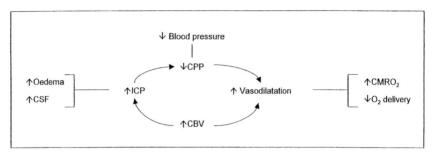

Vasoconstriction cascade

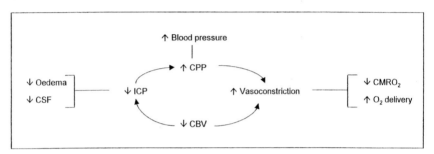

Figure 1.3   The vasoconstrictor and vasodilatory cascades proposed to operate within an intact pressure autoregulatory system, to explain the fall in intracranial pressure following restoration of blood pressure. CBV = cerebral blood volume; CMRO$_2$ = cerebral metabolic rate for oxygen; CPP = cerebral perfusionpressure; CSF = cerebrospinal fluid; ICP = intracranial pressure.

After severe head injury, cerebral autoregulation is disturbed. Animal studies suggest that the lower limit of perfusion pressure at which autoregulation functions is increased.[25] The end result is that a higher than normal CPP is required to ensure global adequacy of cerebral blood flow. It is inevitable, therefore, that the range over which ICP varies directly with CPP also rises to include the blood pressure ranges within which conventional ICP-directed therapies operate. This explains the apparent paralysis of cerebral vessels after head injury.

Practicalities of cerebral perfusion pressure directed therapy

Considerable attention has been focused on the more contentious issues of CPP directed management for head injury, although the basis of the regimen is founded on good general intensive care practice.[15] Inattention to factors that lower blood pressure and hence CPP will be reflected in rises in ICP and the development of ICP pressure waves. In addition to adequate fluid resuscitation, oxygenation and sedation for the head injured patient, there should be a continual assessment of the effects of agents such as mannitol and barbiturates in the light of their potential abilities to worsen an injury by causing hypovolaemia or hypotension. The use of invasive monitoring such as pulmonary artery catheters and daily weight measurement, therefore enables an accurate assessment of the impact of these factors and helps guide their use. Fluid infusions should be chosen based on appropriate haematocrit levels for optimal oxygen carriage and cerebral blood flow.

In addition, therapy is directed at stabilising CPP above the lower autoregulation limit to prevent ICP pressure waves. This has been interpreted as maintaining CPP in excess of 70 mmHg by the use of vasopressors and inotropes. Many critics have pointed to problems of end organ dysfunction in patients managed in this way, particularly concerns about the incidence of adult respiratory distress syndrome (ARDS) and acute renal failure, and the perceived risks of increasing the incidence of secondary intracranial haemorrhage.[26] However, Rosner reported that in 60% of his patients it was possible to ensure an adequate blood pressure and CPP to prevent ICP pressure waves simply by carefully managing fluid balance and sedation.[18] In the remainder of cases, which included those with multisystem trauma, vasopressors such as noradrenaline (norepinephrine) were required, but the incidence of multisystem organ failures was no higher than predicted.

ICP remains an important treatment factor but is no longer the primary treatment goal. A minimum CPP should be determined to ensure that ICP does not vary directly with changes in blood pressure, and is continually reassessed in response to different therapies and over time. Rosner reported a wide variation in this critical level of CPP from 50 to 130 mmHg. Rises in ICP should always be investigated and treated, but in the context of ensuring an adequate CPP. Drainage of CSF and administration of mannitol, both of which have also been shown to be beneficial in reducing ICP, can be used to improve cerebral blood flow. If no identifiable cause can be found for an increased ICP, and CPP appears satisfactory, ICP values above conventional treatment levels are tolerated. This is judged preferable to subjecting patients to therapies that are potentially deleterious, in order to maintain an adequate CPP.

Initial data suggested that CPP directed therapy is beneficial. Patients with a closed head injury and post-resuscitation GCS of less than 7 had an overall mortality of only 30%, compared with 60% mortality in matched historical controls.[18] Importantly, the number of surviving patients with a poor neurological outcome was also reduced. However, the ethical considerations of a true randomised controlled trial remain prohibitive. A recent study carried out by Robertson et al. has attempted to control some of these factors by examining the frequency of jugular venous desaturation in two groups of patients where ICP and CPP were each individually the primary therapeutic target.[26] Although the groups were not exactly similar in other respects, it demonstrated that episodes of desaturation consistent with ischaemia were less frequent in the CPP targeted group.

Problems of CPP directed therapy

The concept of CPP directed therapy has become increasingly popular, although doubts remain as to its applicability in all cases of head injury.[27] There is evidence to support the premise of preservation of cerebral autoregulation to maintain cerebral blood flow, but such a proscriptive regimen may not be appropriate on all occasions. There is little doubt that many treatments aimed at lowering ICP can be detrimental to the brain, particularly in the early resuscitation period.[28] Cerebral ischaemia is most marked within the first 24 hours post-injury, and hypotension compromising CPP is most likely in the first 4 hours.[29] Cerebral metabolism is still high in the first 6 hour period after injury, but cerebral blood flow is likely to be reduced. It has been shown that about a third of patients have globally reduced cerebral blood flow (<18 ml/100 g/min) within 6 hours of injury. Elevation of CPP may therefore be beneficial in ensuring adequacy of cerebral blood flow, and low cerebral blood flows have been shown to be associated with a poor outcome.[30] However, 24 hours after injury, cerebral metabolism decreases, and raising CPP to maximise CBF may constitute overtreatment and may indeed be linked to increased morbidity. Matching CBF to cerebral oxygen extraction may be as beneficial in reducing morbidity as CPP directed therapy. Cruz recently described such a technique using "controlled hyperventilation" guided by jugular bulb oximetry to match flow with global cerebral oxygen extraction, although CPP was maintained above the conventional lower limit of 70 mmHg throughout.[7] In addition, there are clearly differences in the causes of a raised ICP and each of these may need different therapeutic approaches in addition to general measures aimed at avoiding ischaemic insults.[31] This may explain why authors advocating such apparently disparate therapies as controlled hyperventilation and tissue volume regulation (Lund protocol) are also able to report good results for their treatment protocols.[6]

Unresolved issues

The best approach given the lack of clear evidence is perhaps a combination of both ICP and CPP directed therapies in conjunction with the best available cerebral monitoring. There is a danger that CPP directed therapy may appear to be an easy solution to the management of head injury, with the assumption that frequent reassessment of the patient at the bedside is no longer necessary.[32] It is clear that in the early phase of head injury management on the ICU, the aim should be to restore cerebral blood flow to the pressure independent portion of the autoregulation curve. It is also clear that the targeting of any therapy to a "magic number" for either ICP or CPP, without consideration of individual patients' needs, is unsatisfactory, and "adequate" PP may be hard to define.

It is possible that it will never be unequivocally shown that CPP directed therapy results in better survival from head injury than control of ICP alone. Likewise the role of "overtreatment" in morbidity may not be demonstrable. There are inherent difficulties in conducting randomised-controlled trials in patients with neurotrauma, due to both ethical issues and specified treatment policies in different ICUs. This was well demonstrated in a recent multicentre trial of hypothermic therapy, which suffered difficulties in both patient recruitment and unifying treatment strategies between participating centres.[33] A co-ordinated approach to the use of cerebral monitoring and investigation of treatment protocols is lacking in the UK, and although 60% of neurosurgical centres have a dedicated intensive care facility, many patients are managed outside of such specialist units.[2] The difficulties in providing a cohesive approach to treatment are therefore immense.

Summary

In general terms we know that cerebral ischaemia, whether due to hypoxia, hypotension or intracranial hypertension, is associated with a poor outcome after head injury. In addition, cerebral blood flow is initially low and ischaemia is a common occurrence post-injury. Reliance on magic numbers for either ICP or CPP is unhelpful, and flow–metabolism coupling appears to be useful in driving forward the search for improved management strategies. Optimal CPP will vary with both the individual and time, and the much-misused CPP number of 70 mmHg can only be at best a guide figure. It is clear that optimal management of neurotrauma should be based on sound basic intensive care practices. The difficulty lies in knowing which patients to treat aggressively without overtreating them, and at present the monitoring modalities to be able to determine this are lacking. We also have additional difficulties in the UK of ensuring that severely head injured patients are managed in specialist centres where experience can be gained to help determine the way forward.

References

1 Jennett B. Historical perspective on head injury. In: Narayan RK, Wilberger JE, Povlishock JT, eds. *Neurotrauma*. New York: McGraw-Hill, 1996.

2 Matta B, Menon D. Severe head injury in the United Kingdom and Ireland: a survey of practice and implications for management. *Crit Care Med* 1996; **24**: 1743–8.

3 McKeating E, Andrews PJD, Tocher JI, Menon DK. The intensive care of severe head injury: a survey of non-neurosurgical centres in the United Kingdom. *Br J Neurosurg* 1998; **12**: 7–14.11.

4 Marshall LF, Bowers SA. Medical management of head injury. *Clin Neurosurg* 1982; **29**: 312–16.

5 Rosner MJ. Introduction to cerebral perfusion pressure management. *Neurosurg Clin North Am* 1995; **6**: 761–73.

6 Asgeirsson B, Grande PO, Nordstrom CH. A new therapy of post-traumatic brain oedema based on haemodynamic principles for brain volume regulation. *Intensive Care Med* 1994; **20**: 260–7.

7 Cruz J. The first decade of continuous monitoring of jugular bulb oxyhemoglobin saturation: management strategies and clinical outcome. *Crit Care Med* 1998; **26**: 344–51.

8 Shoemaker WC, Appel PL, Kram HB, Waxman K, Lee T-S. Prospective trial of supranormal values of survivors as therapeutic goals in high-risk surgical patients. *Chest* 1988; **94**: 1176–86.

9 Jennett B, Bond M. Assessment of outcome after severe brain damage. *Lancet* 1975; **1**(7905): 480–4.

10 Lang EW, Chesnut RM. Intracranial pressure and cerebral perfusion pressure in severe head injury. *New Horiz* 1995; **3**: 400–9.

11 Marmarou A, Anderson RL, Ward JD. Impact of ICP instability and hypotension on outcome in patients with severe head trauma. *J Neurosurg* 1991; **75** (suppl): S159–66.

12 Langfitt TW, Weinstein JD, Kassell NF. Cerebral vasomotor paralysis produced by intracranial hypertension. *Neurology* 1965; **15**: 622–41.

13 Langfitt TW, Tannanbaum HM, Kassell NF. The etiology of acute brain swelling following experimental head injury. *J Neurosurg* 1966; **24**: 47–56.

14 Becker DP, Miller JD, Ward JD. The outcome from severe head injury with early diagnosis and intensive management. *J Neurosurg* 1977; **47**: 491–502.

15 Chesnut RM. Hyperventilation in traumatic brain injury: friend or foe? *Crit Care Med* 1997; **25**: 1275–8.

16 Changaris DG, McGraw CP, Richardson JD, Garretson HD, Arpin EJ, Shields CB. Correlation of cerebral perfusion pressure and Glasgow Coma Score to outcome. *J Trauma* 1987; **27**: 1007–13.

17 Chan K, Dearden NM, Miller JD. Multimodality monitoring as a guide to treatment of intracranial hypertension after severe brain injury. *Neurosurgery* 1993; **32**: 547–53.

18 Rosner MJ, Rosner SD, Johnson AH. Cerebral perfusion pressure: management protocol and clinical results. *J Neurosurg* 1995; **83**: 949–62.

19 Wolff HG, Forbes HS. Observations on the pial circulation during changes in intracranial pressure. *Arch Neurol Psychol* 1928; **20**: 1035–47.

20 Lundberg N. Continuous recording and control of ventricular fluid pressure in neurosurgical practice. *Acta Psychiatr Scand* 1960; **36** (suppl 149): 1–193.

21 Rosner MJ, Becker DP. Origin and evolution of plateau waves. *J Neurosurg* 1984; **60**: 312–24.
22 Cushing H. Concerning a definite regulatory mechanism of the vasomotor centre which controls blood pressure during cerebral compression. *Bull John Hopkins Hosp* 1901; **12**: 290.
23 Rosner MJ, Newsome HH, Becker DP. Mechanical brain injury: the sympathoadrenal response. *J Neurosurg* 1984; **61**: 76–86.
24 Kontos HA, Wei EP, Navari RM. Responses of cerebral arteries and arterioles to acute hypotension and hypertension. *Am J Physiol* 1978; **234**: H371–83.
25 Lewelt W, Jenkins LW, Miller JD. Autoregulation of cerebral blood flow after experimental fluid percussion injury of the brain. *J Neurosurg* 1980; **53**: 500–11.
26 Robertson CS, Valadka AB, Hannay J et al. Prevention of secondary ischaemic insults after severe head injury. *Crit Care Med* 1999; **27**: 2086–96.
27 Chesnut RM. Medical management of severe head injury: present and future. *New Horiz* 1995; **3**: 581–92.
28 Chesnut RM. Avoidance of hypotension: conditio sine qua non of successful severe head-injury management. *J Trauma* 1997; **42**: S4–9.
29 Bouma GJ, Muizelaar JP, Choi SC, Newlon PG, Young HF. Cerebral circulation and metabolism after severe traumatic brain injury: the elusive role of ischaemia. *J Neurosurg* 1991; **75**: 685–93.
30 Robertson CS, Contant CF, Gokaslan ZL. Cerebral blood flow, arteriovenous oxygen difference, and outcome in head injured patients. *J Neurol Neurosurg Psych* 1992; **55**: 594–603.
31 Miller JD, Piper IR, Dearden NM. Management of intracranial hypertension in head injury: matching treatment with cause. *Acta Neurochir Suppl (Wien)* 1993; **57**: 152–9.
32 Chesnut RM. Guidelines for the management of severe head injury. What we know and what we think we know. *J Trauma* 1997; **42**: S19–22.
33 Anonymous. National Acute Brain Injury Study: *Hypothermia: Performance and Safety Monitoring Board*. 1997.

2: Severe brain insult in the intensive care unit: neurophysiological and clinical assessment of outcome

I ROBERT GHOSH

Introduction

The prediction of outcome after brain insult is a common challenge to all clinicians, most notably the intensive care physician. Increasing numbers of patients are surviving the initial critical event as a direct consequence of improved facilities for immediate resuscitation in the emergency room and intensive care unit (ICU). The cessation of treatment in the setting of potentially reversible brain dysfunction is disastrous, while most would agree that continuing therapy in the face of inevitable brain death is both inhumane and costly. Proper identification of survivors for whom there is no hope of cognitive function is very important, and procrastination by physicians will only add to the family's despair. Furthermore, it is not acceptable for judgements to be based purely on anecdotes or economics. Novel methods of assessment that provide timely and reliable identification of a clear optimistic or pessimistic outlook should be encouraged, while evidence based information for existing methods should be acknowledged and critically assessed. Genuine advances and subsequent changes in practice are infrequent in this difficult area, where most seminal studies date back several years. This review will address the problems associated with the clinical and neurophysiological determination of outcome in patients with severe brain injury.

Problems inherent in predicting outcome after brain injury

There are difficult issues at the outset (Box 2.1). Specific neurological features, for example brain stem areflexia, may have different implications

12

in drug toxicity as compared to traumatic or anoxic brain insult. The medical profession and the public at large need to decide the degree of certainty for poor outlook that is required in order to justify the withdrawal of treatment, as very few scenarios give 100% specificity for non-recovery. Non-brain contributors to illness, for example unstable cardiovascular status, are just as likely to influence outcome as brain injury itself. The reversible sedative component of brain dysfunction is often impossible to quantify. The prediction in an unresponsive patient of longer-term improvement (e.g. the development of higher cognitive functions) is generally impossible, although the prediction of short-term progress such as subsequent responsiveness to physical stimuli is a realistic aim. Finally, if the withdrawal of treatment leads to death, the death itself is often mistakenly accepted as "evidence", thereby validating future treatment withdrawal in similar circumstances. This "self-fulfilling prophecy", although a cliché, is nevertheless correctly highlighted in all debates regarding prognostication.

Box 2.1 Problems in predicting outcome after brain injury

- Different scenarios (e.g. brain stem areflexia) have different implications for different types of brain insult
- Difficulty in the identification of the level of certainty (of poor outlook) required to justify withdrawal of treatment
- Non-brain contributions to outcome
- Influence of sedation on cerebral dysfunction
- Unrealistic attempts to predict long-term outcome

The options

The Glasgow Coma Score (GCS) has been used in the clinical assessment of head injury for many years and is known to correlate well with outcome in this context. When a patient is sedated, artificially ventilated, has multiple severe injuries or has other causes of cerebral dysfunction, the score can be difficult to interpret (or wrongly applied) and an additional method of assessment becomes of paramount clinical importance. There are three main types of assessment of outcome after brain injury. These are neurological examination, electroencephalography (EEG) and evoked potentials (EP). Although studies have extolled the virtues of each of these approaches in isolation, comparisons between them have rarely been comprehensive.

Neurological examination

Comprehensive neurological examinations are not performed frequently in ICUs, under the assumption that there are often no markers to identify deterioration. Although this is occasionally true, the often neglected characteristics that provide prognostic guidance are well documented and include spontaneous eye opening, pupillary light reflex, ciliospinal reflex, oculocephalic and oculovestibular reflexes, motor response to noxious stimuli, spontaneous posturing and respiratory patterns, although the latter is often masked by mechanical ventilation (Box 2.2). These features may be categorised into syndromic patterns in the setting of diffuse traumatic brain injuries and thereby reflect the degree of brain involvement. In ascending order of severity, these are hemispheric, diencephalic, mesencephalopontine, and bulbar (Table 2.1). Hemispheric syndromes carry a better prognosis, while bulbar syndromes are inevitably terminal.[1]

Some additional scenarios have significant implications for outcome. Myoclonus status, which will be discussed later, is an agonal condition post anoxia[2] and after circulatory arrest; there is a defined period beyond which the reappearance of spontaneous respiration, pupillary light reflex, coughing, and ciliospinal reflex are unlikely.[3] However brain stem areflexia after drug intoxication may be reversible within 24 hours.

The first three days are crucial in the determination of outcome in comatose survivors of circulatory arrest.[4] Those patients who do not become brain dead may either recover some degree of awareness or remain in a permanent vegetative state, depending on the degree of cerebral cortical damage. Although clinical examination of cortical function in the early phase of post-anoxic coma is difficult, isolated specific scenarios facilitate prognostication.

Box 2.2   Neurological assessment after brain insult

- Spontaneous eye opening

- Pupillary light reflex

- Ciliospinal reflex

- Oculocephalic/occulovestibular reflexes

- Motor responses to noxious stimulus

- Spontaneous posturing

- Respiratory patterns (may be masked during mechanical ventilation)

Table 2.1 Syndromic patterns and severity of brain injury

Syndromes	Pupils	Eye position	Oculocephalic reflex	Oculovestibular reflex	Tone/posture	Noxious stimulus	Respiration
Hemispheric (cortical/subcortical)	Normal	Normal	Present	Tonic	Paratonic rigidity (forebrain/frontal cortex)	Normal	Cheyne–Stokes (deep hemispheric)
Diencephalic (thalamus/hypothalamus/basal ganglia/internal capsule)	Small, with intact reflexes	Straight ahead or slight divergence	Present	Slow sustained	Paratonic or decorticate rigidity (corticospinal pathways)	Normal or abnormal flexion	
		Complete deviation (ipsilateral to lesion)					
		Slow pendular conjugate movements					
Mesencephalopontine	Pinpoint=pontine	Mid-position irregular= nuclear midbrain	Present	Dysconjugate	Decorticate rigidity	Abnormal flexion= decorticate	Neurogenic hyperventilation (mesencephalic tegmentum)
	Bilateral sight dilatation with intact ciliospinal though no light reflex=pretectal midbrain	Complete ipsilateral deviation	Absent	Absent	Decerebrate rigidity (rostral brain stem and mid pons)	Extension= decerebrate	
	No ciliospinal or light reflex= nuclear midbrain	Slow pendular conjugate movements			Flaccid tetraplegia (ventral pons)		
Bulbar	No ciliospinal reflex	Mid-position	Absent	Absent	Flaccid tetraplegia (medulla)	No response	Irregular, ataxic breathing (medullary)
							Apnoea (severe medullary)

Generalised myoclonus status inevitably results in a permanent vegetative state or death. Myoclonic seizures lack an atonic component and typically involve facial muscles and other axial structures. There are associations with burst suppression on EEG, cerebral oedema or cerebral infarcts on computed tomography (CT) scans, and histopathological evidence of acute ischaemic neuronal change in all cortical laminae. In their study of 107 consecutive patients who remained comatose after cardiac resuscitation, Wijdicks et al.[2] detected myoclonus status in 37%, of whom all died; of the remaining 63% of patients without myoclonus status, 19% awakened. These findings were consistent with earlier reports and confirmed suspicions that myoclonus status in post-anoxic coma indicates devastating neocortical damage, is highly specific for poor cerebral outcome after circulatory arrest, and should therefore influence the decision to withdraw life support. One should note that touch, tracheal suctioning, or loud hand claps can at times trigger single myoclonic jerks; these should be distinguished from myoclonus status or other types of seizures.

Bricolo et al., in their study of 800 patients with acute head injuries, frequently found combinations of extensor and flexor spontaneous posturing and/or responses in the same patient.[5] Each postural constellation had its own distinct neurological signs and prognosis. The incidence of decerebrate rigidity was almost 40%, and in these patients overall survival was markedly reduced though interestingly, good recovery was achieved in 16%, suggesting that extensor motor abnormalities in acute traumatic brain injury do not always reflect poor prognosis.

Electroencephalography and evoked potentials

Those not integrally involved in clinical neurophysiology poorly understand electroencephalograms and evoked potentials. EEGs are electrographic measurements of scalp summated neuronal generated inhibitory and excitatory post-synaptic potentials. They are non-specific, though sensitive, tests of cerebral function and their most frequent use outside the ICU is for confirmation and classification of epilepsy.

In the ICU certain EEG patterns, particularly complete suppression of cortical activity or evolutionary change from mixed activity into burst suppression, have been shown to be highly predictive of poor outcome. The EEG features used to assess the severity of cerebral injury include variability of waveforms and reactivity to various grades of sensory stimuli. Spontaneous pathological changes in the level of arousal, similar to changes in stages of physiological sleep, have been shown in patients with brain damage, and it has been postulated that the absence of these changes signifies a poor outlook.

It is usual for the copious amounts of EEG data to be condensed by processing. Compressed spectral array (frequency analysis),[6] cerebral function analysing monitoring (amplitude analysis),[7] and pattern recognition are some of the commonest processing techniques. The cerebral function analysing monitor (CFAM) is a sophisticated development of the cerebral function monitor (CFM). It produces a condensed analysis of EEG amplitude, analyses the power of the waveform frequencies, and categorises the latter into alpha, beta, theta and delta bands. It can analyse the EEG from two input channels, produce traces of the raw EEG, and incorporate visual, auditory, somatosensory and brain stem evoked potentials.[7] Tools such as these facilitate trend analysis, enable retrospective event detection, and occasionally provide warning devices (especially for seizure detection). Although processed EEGs have been devised to provide increased guidance and independence for the intensive care specialist from the clinical neurophysiologist, she/he needs to be aware that they are not "magic buttons". A basic working knowledge of electroencephalography is essential.

Evoked potentials are cortical action potential responses to sensory (auditory, visual and somatosensory) stimuli. Somatosensory (SSEP) and brain stem (BAEP) evoked potentials are used in the ICU, though less frequently than EEGs as they are probably even less well understood. Although they seem potentially more attractive than EEGs on the basis of practicality, such as a need for fewer scalp electrodes, and importantly, robustness in the face of sedative therapy, the waveforms are much more vulnerable to electrical interference than those of the EEG. Cortical SSEPs, performed within three days, have some predictive value in anoxic brain insult.[8] Although bilaterally absent median nerve SSEPs imply no cerebral recovery, this sign is thought by many to lack sensitivity, as other clinical and electroencephalographic features providing similar implications invariably precede it. Worryingly there have been documented cases of good recovery on rare occasions.[9] Attempts have been made to grade anoxic brain insult using BAEP recordings, though the latter are even more robust than SSEPs; their bilateral absence is associated with established preceding brain stem areflexia. There is interesting ongoing research in the assessment of correlations between BAEP recordings and raised intracranial pressure and also sedation grading.

Polygraphy

Although not routinely performed in clinical practice, many researchers have successfully demonstrated the value of the simultaneous monitoring of EEG with other parameters, for example heart rate and respiratory rate (polygraphic EEG or EEGP). It has been shown that EEGP activity related to sleep is recognisable in the damaged brain and correlates well with the severity of the damage after head injury.[10] This author is presently involved in the clinical and EEGP (EEG, EP, heart rate, skin impedance) evaluation

17

of traumatic, anoxic and toxic/metabolic brain injury, at differing levels of sedation. The attachment of clinical findings to EEGP (EEGP-C) seems to be a logical extension, and is likely to provide more guidance than simply EEG or EEGP.

Sedation

Although the clinical and electrophysiological scenarios and their prognostic implications seem reasonably clear, an unanswered issue for physicians in the ICU is the lack of data that can be extrapolated for concomitant sedation. Therefore, the question "how much is residual sedation contributing to coma?" has not been adequately resolved, either for neurological examination or EEG. This clearly needs addressing, as sedation provides a definite reversible component to cerebral dysfunction. Prospective studies, such as those ongoing at the author's centre, assessing neurological and EEG/EP features at differing levels of sedation in the setting of different types of brain insult, should therefore be encouraged.

"Self-fulfilling prophecy"

In patients with severe systemic or cerebral disease, withdrawal of treatment in response to a postulated poor prognostic sign will often directly lead to death. In this circumstance the *withdrawal of treatment, and not the poor prognostic sign* should be seen as the cause of death. By contrast, if death is perceived as an inevitable consequence of a specific scenario, only then will the latter be considered as having possible prognostic value. Validation is then required in the form of observation in large numbers, or randomized trials of continued treatment versus withdrawal of treatment. Necropsy specimens may help to confirm the extent of brain injury, though one should be certain of the correlation between the pathological findings and the relevant neurological features.

Conclusion

Ongoing research and the accumulation of evidence based information concerning prognostication in brain injury is justified. The problems of assessment, including the quantification of the contribution of sedation, need to be addressed. One needs to be realistic about what can or cannot be predicted on the basis of any assessment. Studies directly comparing different assessment methods should be encouraged. Finally, local and national protocols are desirable in order to provide clear communication between the intensivist and the clinical neurophysiologist; both parties should identify clinical questions that can be answered with the available evidence. It is time to bring the ICU/clinical neurophysiology interface out of the dark ages.

References

1 Bricolo A, Turazzi S, Faccioli F. Combined clinical and EEG examinations for assessment of severity of acute head injuries. *Acta Neurochir* 1979;suppl 28:35–9.
2 Wijdicks EFM, Parisi JE, Sharbrough FW. Prognostic value of myoclonus status in comatose survivors of cardiac arrest. *Ann Neurol* 1994;35:239–43.
3 Jørgensen EO, Malchow-Møller A. Cerebral prognostic signs during cardiopulmonary resuscitation. *Resuscitation* 1978;6:217–25.
4 Levy DE, Caronna JJ, Singer BH, *et al*. Predicting outcome from hypoxic-ischemic coma. *JAMA* 1985;253:1420–6.
5 Brunko E, Zegers de Beyl D. Prognostic value of early cortical somatosensory evoked potentials after resuscitation from cardiac arrest. *Electroencephalogr Clin Neurophysiol* 1987;66:15–24.
6 Bricolo A, Turazzi S, Alexandre A, Rizzuto N. Decerebrate rigidity in acute head injury. *J Neurosurg* 1977;47:680–89.
7 Bickford RG. Newer methods of recording and analyzing EEG. In: Klass DW, Daly DD, eds. *Current practice of clinical electroencephalography*. New York: Raven Press, 1979.
8 Maynard DE, Jenkinson JL. The cerebral function analysing monitor. *Anaesthesia* 1984;39:678–90.
9 Ganes T, Lundar T. EEG and evoked potentials in comatose patients with severe brain damage. *Electroencephalogr Clin Neurophysiol* 1988;69:6–13.
10 Evans BM, Bartlett JR. Prediction of outcome in severe head injury based on recognition of sleep related activity in the polygraphic electroencephalogram. *J Neurol Neurosurg Psychol* 1995;59:17–25.

3: Surgical and radiological treatment of sub-arachnoid haemorrhage

MICHAEL G O'SULLIVAN

Introduction

During the last three decades, new diagnostic techniques and therapeutic strategies have emerged for patients with aneurysmal sub-arachnoid haemorrhage. The introduction of computed tomography (CT) and catheter angiography has improved the accuracy of diagnosis and provided a tool in the evaluation of the clinical course. The application of the operating microscope has refined microsurgical techniques. More recently, the calcium antagonist nimodipine has been shown to improve outcome. Since fluid restriction and the use of antihypertensive drugs have been found to be harmful, hypervolaemia, haemodilution, and in some instances even induced hypertension have been advocated. Moreover, the timing of surgery has shifted for certain categories of patients from late (>10 days) to early (0–3 days) after the initial haemorrhage. Delayed cerebral ischaemia is a major cause of death and disability in patients who initially survive an aneurysmal sub-arachnoid haemorrhage.

The scope of the problem

The pressure within an intracranial aneurysm is equal to the mean arterial blood pressure, which is approximately 80 mmHg. The pressure in the sub-arachnoid space is approximately 10 mmHg, such that the cerebral perfusion pressure in the brain (or across the wall of the aneurysm) is about 70 mmHg. When an aneurysm ruptures, there is a fistula between the intravascular circulation and the CSF circulation so that the intracranial pressure (ICP) suddenly increases. If the ICP is equal to the mean arterial blood pressure the cerebral perfusion pressure (CPP) is zero, which means that cerebral blood flow is also zero. If this scenario lasts about 10 seconds unconsciousness will occur and death occurs within about 3 minutes. It is estimated that about 20% of patients with sub-arachnoid haemorrhage die at ictus. Of those who survive another 15% die within the following 24 hours, despite optimum medical care. Overall, the outcome is favourable in only 40% of patients who survive to reach hospital. Sub-arachnoid haemorrhage is clearly a devastating and very often fatal illness. Although the major cause of morbidity and mortality after sub-arachnoid haemorrhage is undoubtedly brain injury caused by the initial bleed, those patients who reach hospital are at risk of several complications, including re-bleeding, cerebral vasospasm (delayed ischaemic neurological deficit), and hydrocephalus. This review will describe the history of the therapeutic strategies that have been used to address these complications.

Re-bleeding

It was previously thought that the highest risk for re-bleeding after sub-arachnoid haemorrhage was between days 7 and 14, when it was presumed re-bleeding occurred due to dissolving of the blood clot sealing the hole in the aneurysm. It is now known that that this is incorrect. Figure 4.1 shows the probability of re-bleeding during the first few days after a sub-arachnoid haemorrhage.[1] It is clear that in fact the highest risk period for re-bleeding is the first 24 hours with a risk of 4%. There is a 60% chance of death with each episode of re-bleeding. Norman Dott, the first Professor of Neurosurgery in Edinburgh, had an interest in sub-arachnoid haemorrhage. In 1931 Dott performed the first craniotomy for a ruptured aneyrusm, wrapping it with muscle. The patient survived in good condition for a further 10 years. Two other patients, however, succumbed, and by 1932 he had abandoned the intracranial procedure in favour of carotid ligation. He expounded on the indications and contraindictions of carotid ligation, which are still valid today. In 1936 Walter Dandy of the Johns Hopkins Hospital performed the first clip ligation of an intracranial aneurysm, which presented with a third nerve palsy.

Thirty years later Gazi Yasargil, of Turkish descent but who worked in Zurich, introduced the operating microscope to neurosurgery; this had dual benefits of illumination and magnification. In conjunction with being a gifted surgeon he also described microneurosurgical anatomy and developed microinstrumentation, which revolutionised the practice of vascular microneurosurgery, such that by 1990 such operations were being performed on even the most elderly and sickest of patients.

In 1990 a new technique devised by Dr Guido Guglieimi, an Italian neuroradiologist, was introduced.[2] The so-called "GDC"–Guglieimi detachable coils – utilises flexible microcatheters which can be pushed and steered into the aneurysm via the femoral artery. Very fine platinum coils

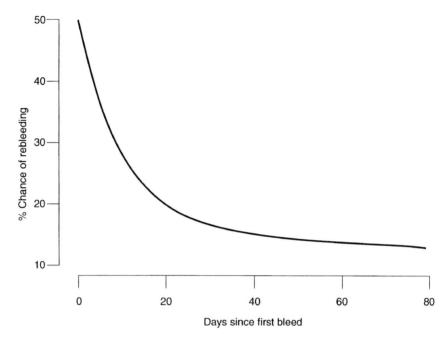

*Figure 4.1   The relationship between the interval from the day of first sub-arachnoid haemorrhage and the chance of re-bleeding. The rate of re-bleeding after 6 months is approximately 3% per year. Reproduced with permission from Jane JA, Kassel NF, Torner JC, et al. J Neurosurg 1985;**62**:321–3.[1]*

can then be delivered into the aneurysm via the microcather. The great advantage of these coils is that they can be withdrawn and repositioned until a good position is achieved before final detachment. The coils are available in variable diameters and lengths and are incredibly fine and soft. The microcatheter is pushed into the aneurysm, through the anterior communicating artery. The coil can then be passed up through the catheter and into the aneurysm. Three dimensional coils are used to form a basket, which occludes the lumen. The basket is then filled up with smaller and smaller coils until the aneurysm is occluded, without ever opening the patient's head.

After several hundred coiling procedures some conclusions can be drawn. Successful GDC obliteration confers short term protection to aneurysm re-bleeding, but because the coils have only been available since 1990 the long term outcome remains unclear. There is a significant failure rate and fatal rupture during surgery occurs in about one in 300 patients.

Timing of surgery

The risk of re-bleeding after a sub-arachnoid haemorrhage is highest in the first 24 hours after haemorrhage. If the highest risk is early on then the sooner patients are operated on the better. Early surgery reduces re-bleeding but it is difficult and has a higher mortality and morbidity because of the difficult conditions under which the operation is performed. If coiling rather than clipping the aneurysm is used, this does not apply because the "surgery" is carried out without opening the patient's head. In Edinburgh 66% of aneurysms are treated by clipping or coiling within three days.

Delayed ischaemic neurological deficit (vasospasm)

Delayed ischaemic neurological deficit is the clinical manifestation of vasospasm, or more accurately, angiographic arterial narrowing, which can be defined as an exaggerated prolonged constriction of blood vessels in response to a sub-arachnoid haemorrhage.[3] Angiographic arterial narrowing occurs in 70% of patients with sub-arachnoid haemorrhage, but not all of these patients are symptomatic. There is no correlation between the presence of angiographic arterial narrowing and symptoms of delayed ischaemic neurological deficit. Transcranial Doppler has shown that when velocity in the middle cerebral artery is more than 120 cm/s, then vasospasm can be demonstrated. However, many patients have high velocities but no symptoms. In the study by Meyer *et al.*, cerebral blood flow after sub-arachnoid haemorrhage was measured (Figure 4.2). The study showed that cerebral blood flow dipped at day 4, remaining low until day 20.[4] The progression of the clinical syndrome mirrors these findings, suggesting an ischaemic deficit. The clinical syndrome of delayed ischaemic neurological deficit occurs predominantly between 4 and 14 days after the haemorrhage and is manifest by deteriorating consciousness with no evidence of re-bleeding, hydrocephalus, or metabolic upset.[5]

Current management recommendations

Many patients with sub-arachnoid haemorrhage develop hyponatraemia, which may be interpreted as inappropriate antidiuretic hormone (ADH) release in association with cerebral salt wasting syndrome. Historically, treatment of ruptured sub-arachnoid aneurysm included fluid restriction and strict control of blood pressure. However fluid restriction is not appropriate, because such treatment may result in an excessive number of

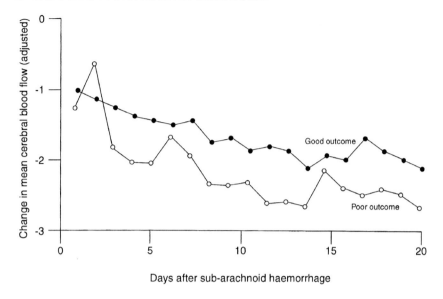

Figure 4.2 Change in mean cerebral blood flow (adjusted for age) after sub-arachnoid haemorrhage in relation to clinical outcome. Good outcome = patients fully employed, no residual symptoms; poor outcome = alive but not fully employable due to residual symptoms. Adapted Meyer CH, Lowe D, Meyer M, Richardson PL, Neil-Dwyer G. Neurosurgery *1983;12:58–76.*[4]

patients developing strokes. If patients are in sodium deficit, sodium repletion may be warranted and in fact the incidence of stroke in these circumstances is much less. It is now known that the sodium natriuresis arises from excessive atrial natiuretic factor release and these patients are indeed hypovolaemic.[6] It is also recommended that all patients are treated with the calcium antagonist nimodipine after sub-arachnoid haemorrhage. Vasospasm may result from the effects of various vasoactive agents in the CSF, leading to an increase of calcium in vascular smooth muscle cells and hence vasoconstriction. A recent study showed a reduction in risk of stroke of 34% when nimodipine 60 mg orally every 4 hours for 21 days is given.[7]

In the study by Origatano[8] a protocol for prophylactic hypertensive hypervolaemic haemodilution ("triple-H" therapy) was investigated for the treatment of sub-arachnoid haemorrhage, and the response of cerebral blood flow was evaluated. Surgery was performed where possible within 24 hours of sub-arachnoid haemorrhage. Cerebral blood flow remained elevated during the 21 days after sub-arachnoid haemorrhage, irrespective of neurological grade on admission, age, sex, or angiographic arterial narrowing. All patients managed with the protocol remained neurologically stable or improved. This study showed that triple-H therapy is safe and effective, and in combination with early aneurysm surgery it can minimise delayed cerebral ischaemia and improve outcome. Many patients are managed with a customised version of the rather extreme protocol advocated by Origatano. Patients are treated initially with hypervolaemia, followed by haemodilution and only have induced hypertension if they are still deteriorating.

Interventional treatment for vasospasm

Some patients who suffer sub-arachnoid haemorrhage develop progressive neurological deficit despite the best medical management including nimodipine and triple-H therapy. Angiographic arterial narrowing can be treated using selective intra-arterial papaverine to improve perfusion. However in many patients a good angiographic picture may not represent clinical improvement and patients do not improve. Narrowing in the internal carotid artery can also be treated by balloon angioplasty, although ruptures can occur and this technique too remains unproven.

Hydrocephalus

Hydrocephalus can be classed as acute, sub-acute, or chronic. In an intensive care setting acute hydrocephalus is seen predominantly. Radiologically, 19% of scans show hydrocephalus within 72 hours of sub-arachnoid haemorrhage
radiographic hydrocephalus. Of these patients 28% are asymptomatic and do not have a depressed level of consciousness. Of those patients who do have a depressed level of consciousness, half improve spontaneously. Symptomatic hydrocephalus with a depressed level of consciousness and obviously enlarged ventricles on CT scan may benefit from treatment. The treatment of choice recommended up until recently was external ventricular drainage of CSF through a ventriculostomy. However, there are two problems with this technique. Infection can be introduced leading to ventriculitis, but more importantly, the risk of re-bleeding is increased. This is because when the consciousness level is depressed, and hydrocephalus is present, it is assumed that intracranial pressure is high, which keeps the aneurysm sealed. If CSF is suddenly lost, intracranial pressure will also suddenly drop and the transmural pressure across the aneurysm will suddenly increase, thus increasing the risk of re-bleeding. It is therefore preferable to treat patients conservatively. An ICP monitor can be inserted and if the pressure increases then this can be followed by ventricular

drainage.

Neurological grading

There has always been a problem with grading neurological severity after sub-arachnoid haemorrhage. Grade 1 can be defined as fully alert, Grade 2 is Glasgow Coma Score (GCS) 13 or 14, Grade 3 is GCS 13–14 plus focal signs such as hemiplegia, Grade 4, GCS 7–12, and Grade 5, GCS 2–6. Grades 1 and 2 are "good" grades and grades 3–5 are "poor" grades. However the timing of grading has remained controversial. A retrospective paper published in 1996 investigated the management of poor grade patients after sub-arachnoid haemorrhage and the importance of radiological findings on clinical outcome.[9] Patients were divided into three groups, depending on whether they had a depressed level of consciousness due to haematoma, hydrocephalus, or just diffuse sub-arachnoid haemorrhage. Poor grade was defined as GCS of 12 or less recorded within the first 24 hours of hospitalisation. The study showed that patients in poor grade due to haematoma had a very poor outcome while patients in poor grade due to sub-arachnoid haemorrhage or hydrocephalus had a favourable outcome in over 50% of cases.

A recent prospective study in Edinburgh including 166 good grade (GCS more than 12) patients over a three year period showed a favourable outcome, defined as a good recovery, or moderately disabled in 90%. Sixteen patients had a poor outcome, which was procedure related in almost half of these, due to non-preventable re-bleeding in five patients and delayed ischaemic deficit in three.

In spite of everything, however, the fatality rate has remained unchanged since 1977. Nearly 40% of patients suffering sub-arachnoid haemorrhage still die. Optimum treatment of sub-arachnoid haemorrhage still has a long way to go, particularly with poor grade patients. It also remains unclear as to the relative benefit of coiling versus clipping. This will hopefully be answered by the results of the International Sub-arachnoid Aneurysm Trial (ISAT).

References

1 Jane JA, Kassel NF, Torner JC, et al. The natural history of aneurysms and arteriovenous malformations. *J Neurosurg* 1985;**62**:321–3.

2 Guglielmi G, Vinuela F, Dion J, et al. Electrothrombosis of saccular aneurysms via endovascular approach. Part 2: Preliminary clinical experience. *J Neurosurg* **75**:8–14.

3 Weir B, MacDonald L. Cerebral vasospasm. *Clin Neurosurg* 1992;**40**:40–55.

4 Meyer CH, Lowe D, Meyer M, Richardson PL, Neil-Dwyer G. Progressive change in cerebral blood flow during the first three weeks after subarachnoid hemorrhage. *Neurosurg* 1983;**12**:58–76.

5 Bervall U, Steiner L, Forster DMC. Early pattern of cerebral circulatory disturbances following subarachnoid haemorrhage. *Neuroradiol* 1973;**5**:24–32.

6 Maroon JC, Nelson PB. Hypovolemia in patients with sub-arachnoid hemorrhage: therapeutic implications. *Neurosurg* 1979;**4**:223–6.

7 Pickard JD, Murray GD, Illingworth R, *et al.* Effect of oral nimodipine on cerebral infarction and outcome after subarachnoid haemorrhage: British aneurysm nimopidpine trial. *Br Med J* 1989;**298**:636–42.

8 Origitano TC, Wascher TM, Reichman OH, Anderson DE. Sustained increased cerebral blood flow with prophylactic hypertensive hypervolemic hemodilution ('triple-H' therapy) after subarachnoid hemorrhage. *Neurosurg* 1990;**27**:729–40.

9 O'Sullivan MG, Sellar R, Statham PF, Whittle IR. Management of poor grade patients after subarachnoid haemorrhage: the importance of neuroradiological findings on clinical outcome. *Br J Neurosurg* 1996;**10**:445–52.

4: Medical management of complications following aneurysmal sub-arachnoid haemorrhage

PETER JD ANDREWS

Introduction

Sub-arachnoid haemorrhage after spontaneous rupture of an aneurysm occurs in 12 per 10 000 people. Of these, 15% will die before they reach hospital and almost 50% die later. Of the survivors, 25% are disabled. The typical age range is 35-60 years, and it occurs more frequently in women than men (Box 3.1). This review will address the medical management of patients who are admitted to the intensive care unit (ICU) with complications following aneurysmal sub-arachnoid haemorrhage. It will focus primarily on cardiac, pulmonary and metabolic complications, but will also mention delayed neurological deficit. It is still not entirely clear whether delayed neurological deficit is due to a failure of oxygen delivery

---

Box 3.1   Sub-arachnoid haemorrhage: facts and figures

- Occurs in 12 per 10 000 population

- 15% die before reaching hospital

- 50% die in hospital

- 25% are permanently disabled

- Age of onset 35–60 years

- Two-thirds are women

---

caused by narrowing of the cerebral arterial vessels as has been assumed. Clinically there is an increase in transcranial Doppler velocities, angiographic arterial vessel narrowing, and a reduction in consciousness. Recent research has also demonstrated that it is possible to monitor impending neurological deficit in the ICU setting and this will be discussed.

The importance of medical complications after sub-arachnoid haemorrhage

In 1995 the Co-operative Aneurysm study was published, providing a unique resource. It was a randomised controlled trial of all grades of patient with sub-arachnoid haemorrhage, such that more than half of the patients were classified as good grade (WFNS I&II). Patients were randomised to receive either the calcium antagonist nicardipine or placebo. This meant that more than 450 patients received no medication, providing a control group for the study of the medical complications after sub-arachnoid haemorrhage including the effect of neurosurgical and neurological critical care interventions and the relationship of those interventions and outcome.[1] Of the 457 patients, of all grades of sub-arachnoid haemorrhage, almost half had vasospasm, re-bleeding occurred in 7% and the three month mortality rate was 19%. Forty per cent of the patients had at least one life threatening medical complication. What is important is that the proportion of deaths from medical complications was almost equal to the mortality

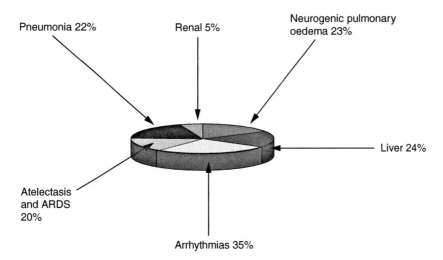

Pneumonia 22%

Renal 5%

Neurogenic pulmonary oedema 23%

Liver 24%

Atelectasis and ARDS 20%

Arrhythmias 35%

Figure 3.1 Pie chart showing the relative percentages of medical complications after aneurysmal sub-arachnoid haemorrhage. Reproduced with permission from Solenski NJ, Haley EC Jr, Kassell NF, et al. Medical complications of aneurysmal subarachnoid hemorrhage: a report of the multicenter, cooperative aneurysm study. Crit Care Med 1995;23:1007–17.[1]

from re-bleeding, the effect of the initial haemorrhage, and vasospasm alone. Thus medical complications do contribute enormously to the morbidity and mortality of sub-arachnoid haemorrhage (Figure 3.1).

Cardiac abnormalities and pulmonary oedema

Life threatening cardiac arrhythmias best describes the electrocardiogram (ECG) changes that occur following sub-arachnoid haemorrhage. Specifically this includes Q wave inversion and prolongation of the QTc interval. In the Co-operative Aneurysm study,[1] 23% of the control patients developed pulmonary oedema, but there was no relationship between the development of pulmonary oedema and so-called triple H therapy (see Chapter 3). Many studies have investigated the ability of ECG changes to predict those patients who go on to develop cardiac and pulmonary complications after sub-arachnoid haemorrhage. In a cohort of all grades of sub-arachnoid haemorrhage patients, ECG changes were used to try and identify those patients who might have left ventricular wall motion disturbance on echocardiography.[2] Fifty-seven patients without any evidence of pre-existing cardiac disease had serial ECGs and echocardiography undertaken. Ventricular wall motion abnormalities were found in only 8%. Interestingly, hypotension and pulmonary oedema were only found in patients who had wall motion defects. The ECG changes that were associated with this were Q wave inversion and prolongation of the QTc segment. The pathophysiology for the cardiac dysfunction may be related to ventricular depolarization, since this is sensitive to high levels of circulatory catecholamines and there were also borderline CKMB elevations in those patients. In addition there was a strong association with poor neurological grade and ECG abnormalities.

The implications of cardiac and pulmonary morbidity have lead to a focus on cardiac morbidity. However later studies show that morbidity or mortality directly linked to cardiac causes is small. A recent study investigated the cardiac related mortality in all grades of patients with sub-arachnoid haemorrhage who had ECG changes consistent with ischaemic or myocardial infarction.[3] Almost 480 patients were studied and 58 fulfilled the criteria for ischaemia or myocardial infarction. Of the 58, 41 were treated neurosurgically, and in this group no deaths resulting from cardiac causes were found. However, 20 of the 58 patients who had EGC changes died. Multivariate analysis showed that age over 65 years and poor grade were the only predictors of mortality. ECG changes, specifically Q wave inversion and ST segment elevation or depression, were not significantly predictive. The authors concluded that the risk of death from cardiac causes is low, with or without neurosurgical intervention, and that ECG abnormalities are associated with more severe neurological injury but are not predictive of all cause mortality.[3]

Cardiogenic shock after sub-arachnoid haemorrhage

A syndrome of severe but reversible left ventricular dysfunction and cardiogenic shock associated with sub-arachnoid haemorrhage has been clearly described[4,5] and which readily responds to dobutamine.[6] Catecholamine release has been suggested as a possible mechanism. When an intracranial aneurysm ruptures, intracranial pressure reaches mean arterial pressure and cerebral perfusion pressure becomes zero. Hopefully reperfusion is established relatively quickly and the physiological response to this is a sympathetic discharge of catecholamines and vasopressin, and this may result in myocardial stunning (Box 3.2).

Box 3.2   Cardiorespiratory dysfunction after sub-arachnoid haemorrhage: mechanisms

● Massive sympathetic discharge

● Catecholamine release

● Systemic to pulmonary circulation shift

● Increased pulmonary permeability

● Myocardial "stunning"

The known effects of β- and α-adrenergic adrenoreceptor agonists can explain the shifting of circulating volume from systemic to pulmonary circulation, increased pulmonary hydrostatic pressure leading to leakage of fluid into the lungs, and the onset of neurogenic pulmonary oedema (Figure 3.2). There is evidence from clinical studies that a hydrostatic mechanism is important in the development of neurogenic pulmonary oedema. Measurement of the protein content in pulmonary alveolar fluids in comparison to the protein content in plasma, at the onset of neurogenic pulmonary oedema, enables the classification of hydrostatic or permeability oedema, depending on protein ratio. Neurogenic pulmonary oedema has been shown to be primarily hydrostatic in origin,[7] supporting the theory of a catecholamine surge with increased pulmonary artery pressure and deranged permeability.

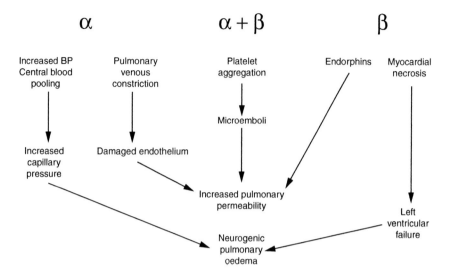

Figure 3.2   Diagram showing the action of α- and β-adrenergic agonists after sub-arachnoid haemorrhage, and how these actions may result in neurogenic pulmonary oedema.

Prediction of cardiac and pulmonary problems

Can cardiogenic shock, neurogenic pulmonary oedema and cardiac dysrrythmia complicating sub-arachnoid haemorrhage be predicted? QTc dispersion on ECG has been used to predict cardiorespiratory compromise.[8] Poor grade sub-arachnoid haemorrhage patients admitted to the ICU were studied. ECG was performed within 24 hours of the onset of sub-arachnoid haemorrhage, before therapy with inotropes was commenced. A simple ECG scoring system was used, where a single point was assigned if any of the key features on ECG were noted (Box 3.3). Those patients who went on to develop cardiorespiratory depression, defined as a requirement for inotropic support (dopamine, adrenaline (epinephrine), dobutamine, or noradrenaline (norepinephrine)), or respiratory compromise (Pao_2/Fio$_2$ ratio ≤40 kPa) were also recorded. The results showed that even in patients who have no EGC abnormalities using the simple scoring system, QTc dispersion was elevated to greater than 50 ms (Figure 3.3) and was different when compared to five ICU control patients, who were in the ICU but not receiving inotropes. There were no differences between the simple ECG score in sub-arachnoid haemorrhage patients and control ICU patients not receiving inotropes, and no effect of age. The control patients and sub-arachnoid haemorrhage patients had

---

Box 3.3   ECG abnormalities

- Heart rate

- Heart rhythm

- Axis

- Block

- P wave

- QRS

- ST segment

- T wave changes

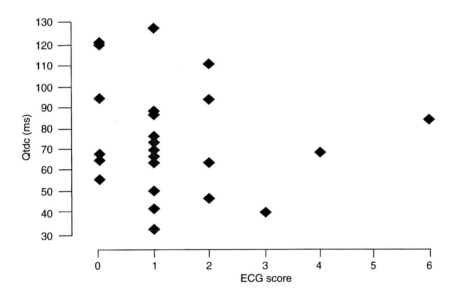

Figure 3.3   Relationship between simple ECG score on admission (see Box 3.3) and QTc dispersion interval (QTdc) in patients admitted to the ICU after sub-arachnoid haemorrhage. See text for details.

different QTc dispersions, and QTc interval was also able to predict cardiorespiratory depression (Figure 3.4). This study demonstrates that QTc interval may be the most sensitive admission ECG abnormality able to predict subsequent development of cardiorespiratory depression by assessing ventricular repolarisation variability.

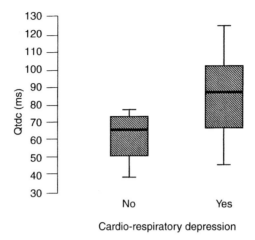

Figure 3.4 Admission ECG QTc dispersion interval (QTdc) in relation to subsequent development of cardiorespiratory depression in patients admitted to the ICU after sub-arachnoid haemorrhage. See text for details.

Delayed neurological deficit

Sub-arachnoid haemorrhage is defined as blood in the sub-arachnoid space but an important feature in aneurysmal sub-arachnoid haemorrhage is that the blood is oxygenated. This is particularly important in relation to late neurological deficit. Although it is clear that something related to the oxyhaemoglobin content of the CSF is causing arterial constriction and hence neurological deficit, it is still not known what exactly causes the arterial narrowing.

How can delayed neurological deficit after sub-arachnoid haemorrhage be monitored and even predicted? Patients in the ICU following sub-arachnoid haemorrhage commonly have pulmonary artery catheters in place, and a whole myriad of monitoring to measure oxygen delivery to the brain, including tissue Po_2 electrodes and jugular bulb oxygen saturation monitors (Figure 3.5). This approach reflects the hypothesis that the delayed neurological deficit is a failure of cellular oxygen delivery caused by arterial vessel narrowing. Of course, patients in the ICU are sedated and a reliable Glasgow Coma Score to assess clinically the degree of neurological dysfunction is not feasible. What is really required is an early warning system to show impending onset before established irreversible cerebral infarction occurs, and without the need for a Glasgow Coma Score. Continuous quantitative EEG monitoring of relative alpha frequencies has been used in this manner.[9] In health the

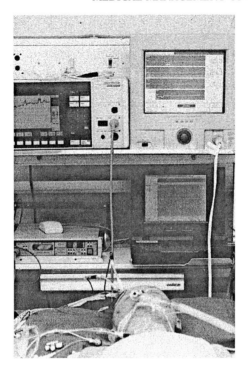

Figure 3.5   Monitoring a patient on the ICU after sub-arachnoid haemorrhage.

cortical rhythm is usually a slow rhythm, superimposed by faster rhythms from brain stem and diencephalon pace makers. It was hypothesised that if dysfunction due to developing delayed neurological deficit occurred this would result in failure of conduction of these pacemaker rhythms from deeper brain stem centres, which would be seen as a reduction in relative alpha frequency. An eight-electrode bipolar longitudinal montage approach was investigated in patients after sub-arachnoid haemorrhage. The relationship of alpha frequency to the percentage of all other frequencies was studied, along with transcranial Doppler velocity, cerebral blood flow using xenon (^{133}Xe), and angiography. Nineteen of 32 patients studied had vasospasm demonstrated by either elevated transcranial Doppler velocities or angiography, and 15 of these had a reduction in relative alpha frequency variability. But, importantly, the reduction in relative alpha frequency occurred in advance of the transcranial Doppler and angiographic changes.[9] In some patients EEG showed a reduction in the alpha frequency without angiographic vessel narrowing or increased transcranial Doppler velocity. However all these patients subsequently developed neurological complications such as raised ICP, re-bleeding, hemiplegia, or embolic stroke. These data suggest that the technique may provide a sensitive monitor of developing neurological deficit that is particularly useful in sedated patients.

Treatment of delayed neurological deficit

Systemic therapy for delayed neurological deficit includes the use of calcium antagonists, triple H therapy, local management of arterial vessel narrowing through angioplasty or papavarine injection and, more recently, intrathecal administration of the nitric oxide donor SNP was used in three patients, with successful reversal of arterial vessel narrowing.[10] In the past many vasodilatory agents have been used to treat arterial vessel narrowing, many of them given systemically in an attempt to achieve high enough concentrations in the cerebral circulation to reverse the vasospasm. Inevitably, the systemic effect, hypotension, due to systemic vasodilatation, resulted in the studies being stopped.

A large meta-analysis of calcium antagonist trials in patients with sub-arachnoid haemorrhage was undertaken[11] to evaluate the results of trials of nimodipine, nicardipine, and the research compound AT877. Ten trials in total were included in the meta-analysis, with data from almost 3000 patients. The overall relative risk reduction was 16% and the relative risk reduction in case fatality was 10% overall. Delayed neurological deficit was reduced by 30% and CT scan documented cerebral infarction was reduced by 20% by the use of calcium antagonists. When nimodipine trials alone were analysed, there was a greater relative risk reduction than with the two other calcium antagonist trials. Interestingly, the research compound AT877 and nicardipine were more effective at reversing angiographically proven arterial vessel narrowing than nimodipine, but were less effective at preventing delayed neurological deficit.

There have been two large randomised studies of tirilazad mesylate, one in North America and one in the United Kingdom, Europe and Australasia. Strangely, the studies produced quite opposite results: in the American study there was no improvement in functional recovery with tirilazad after sub-arachnoid haemorrhage.[12] However, in the study in the UK, Europe and Australasia, there was an improvement in the patients treated with tirilazad, but this was restricted to male patients.[13] Pharmacokinetic studies revealed that tirilazad is metabolised more rapidly in women than men. As two-thirds of the patients who have sub-arachnoid haemorrhage are women, it is surprising that closer attention was not paid to pharmacokinetic differences between the sexes before the study was undertaken. However with redesigned dosing schedules this therapy may be useful in the future.

Intravascular volume depletion and hyponatraemia

One other feature of sub-arachnoid haemorrhage is intravascular volume depletion and loss of sodium. A recent study investigated the use of 5% albumin on sodium balance after sub-arachnoid haemorrhage.[14] Patients were randomised to receive saline plus 5% albumin to either a normal perfusion cardiovascular pressure (CVP) (≤5 mmHg, normovolaemic group) or to a CVP of ≥8 mmHg (hypervolaemic group). The hypervolaemic group received significantly more fluid, albumin, and sodium. Cumulative sodium balance was persistently negative in the normovolaemic group because of losses occurring on days 2 and 3, but not in the hypervolaemic group. The mechanism remains unclear, and, paradoxically, those patients who were given more fluid resuscitation and more 5% albumin actually had a lower glomerular filtration rate.[14]

Conclusion

In conclusion, the proportion of deaths from a medical complication following sub-arachnoid haemorrhage is equal to that from either direct effects of the haemorrhage, re-bleeding or vasospasm individually. Pulmonary complications are the most common non-neurological cause of death. Although there have been several promising studies of both monitoring techniques and potential therapeutic strategies, calcium antagonists and supportive approaches may still be the best we can offer at present.

References

1 Solenski NJ, Haley EC Jr, Kassell NF, *et al.* Medical complications of aneurysmal subarachnoid hemorrhage: a report of the multicenter, cooperative aneurysm study. *Crit Care Med* 1995;**23**:1007–17.
2 Mayer SA, LiMandri G, Sherman D, *et al.* Electrocardiographic markers of abnormal left ventricular wall motion in acute subarachnoid hemorrhage. *J Neurosurg* 1995;**83**:889–96.
3 Zaroff JG, Rordorf GA, Newell JB, Ogilvy CS, Levinson JR. Cardiac outcome in patients with subarachnoid hemorrhage and electrocardiographic abnormalities. *Neurosurg* 1999;**44**:34–40.
4 Wells C, Cujec B, Johnson D, Goplen G. Reversibility of severe left ventricular dysfunction in patients with subarachnoid hemorrhage. *Am Heart J* 1995;**129**:409–12.
5 Parr MJ, Finfer SR, Morgan MK. Reversible cardiogenic shock complicating subarachnoid haemorrhage. *Br Med J* 1996;**313**:681–3.

6 Deehan SC, Grant IS. Haemodynamic changes in neurogenic pulmonary oedema: effect of dobutamine. *Intensive Care Med* 1996;**22:**672–6.
7 Smith WS, Matthay MA. Evidence for a hydrostatic mechanism in human neurogenic pulmonary edema. *Chest* 1997;**111:**1326–33.
8 MacMillan CSA, Andrews PJD, Struthers AD. Acute brain injury and the ECG: QT dispersion is increased. *Br J Anaesth* 1998;**81:**819P (abstract).
9 Vespa PM, Nuwer MR, Juhasz C, *et al.* Early detection of vasospasm after acute subarachnoid hemorrhage using continuous EEG ICU monitoring. *Electroencephalogr Clin Neurophysiol* 1997;**103:**607–15.
10 Thomas JE, Rosenwasser RH, Selman WR, *et al.* Reversal of severe cerebral vasospasm in three patients after aneurysmal subarachnoid hemorrhage: initial observations regarding the use of intraventricular sodium nitroprusside in humans. *Neurosurg* 1999;**44:**48–58.
11 Feigin VL, Rinkel GJ, Algra A, Vermeulen M, van Gijn J. Calcium antagonists in patients with aneurysmal subarachnoid hemorrhage: a systematic review. *Neurology* 1998;**50:**876–83.
12 Haley ECJ, Kassell NF, Apperson-Hansen C, Maile MH, Alves WM. A randomized, double-blind, vehicle-controlled trial of tirilazad mesylate in patients with aneurysmal subarachnoid hemorrhage: a cooperative study in North America. *J Neurosurg* 1997;**86:**467–74.
13 Kassell NF, Haley EC Jr, Apperson-Hansen C, Alves WM. Randomized, double-blind, vehicle-controlled trial of tirilazad mesylate in patients with aneurysmal subarachnoid hemorrhage. A cooperative study in Europe, Australia, and New Zealand. *J Neurosurg* 1996;**84:**221–8.
14 Mayer SA, Solomon RA, Fink ME, *et al.* Effect of 5% albumin solution on sodium balance and blood volume after subarachnoid hemorrhage. *Neurosurg* 1998;**42:**759–68.

5: Sub-arachnoid haemorrhage: case presentation

GRAHAM R NIMMO

This chapter provides an example of a case of aneurysmal sub-arachnoid haemorrhage and attempts to highlight some of the problems of the intensive care unit (ICU) management of this type of patient.

Presentation

The case presented is a young Scottish woman aged 32. She had been unwell for a couple of days. There has been some mention in the literature of headaches and pre-bleeds prior to a sub-arachnoid haemorrhage, and some patients have described this type of experience before the onset of haemorrhage. This particular lady had had some degree of neck stiffness. She had collapsed in the bathroom about 20 minutes after intercourse and was found by her husband. She was taken into accident and emergency and at that point was agitated with a Glasgow Coma Score (GCS) of 9 and no focal neurology. Her blood pressure was slightly elevated at 160/90 mmHg, heart rate 80/min, and respiratory rate 18/min. Tachycardia and hypertension are both commonly seen as a result of catecholamine release after sub-arachnoid haemorrhage.

At this stage she was anaesthetised, paralysed, intubated and ventilated for transfer for computed tomography (CT) scan. The aim of anaesthesia in these cases is to provide satisfactory conditions for intubation and ventilation while avoiding either hypotension or hypertension. Occasionally patients with a low GCS have been laryngoscoped and intubated without anaesthesia, which can result in re-bleeding. This patient became slightly hypotensive (BP 95/60 mmHg) after anaesthesia and was given volume loading with colloid before being transferred for CT scan.

The CT scan demonstrated the presence of blood in the sub-arachnoid space, generally settled in the ventricles, with a predominance of blood in the posterior fossa. An intracranial pressure (ICP) monitor was inserted and the patient's ICP was normal at this stage, at 6 mmHg. She was still rather hypotensive but with a very good cerebral perfusion pressure (CPP) of 74 mmHg.

Central venous and jugular lines were inserted and interestingly the jugular venous oxygen saturation was extremely low (25%), suggesting a very high cerebral metabolic rate or a very low cerebral oxygen delivery. Pao_2 was 17.1 kPa, $Paco_2$ was 3.7 kPa on 40% inspired oxygen. A reduction in minute ventilation to increase $Paco_2$ was therefore instituted and nasogastric nimodipine was commenced. Within a few hours the jugular venous oxygen saturation had increased to 53%. Sedation was reduced for neurological assessment, the patient was opening her eyes and flexing her arms and legs, with an improvement in GCS from presentation. She therefore proceeded to angiography and coiling of the posterior inferior communicating artery aneurysm. She was heparinised although this is not universal practice following coiling.

Day 2

By 1 o'clock the next morning, nearly 24 hours after presentation, the patient had a Pao_2 of about 14 kPa on 100% oxygen and her mean arterial blood pressure was 65 mmHg.

A chest X-ray showed pulmonary oedema. It should be remembered that neurogenic pulmonary oedema may commonly occur in patients with ischaemic brain and high ICP, pulmonary oedema may recur. Neurogenic pulmonary oedema is normally a low protein, high permeability hydrostatic type of pulmonary oedema. Although that is generally true, there are some patients who have had sub-arachnoid haemorrhage who develop an acute respiratory distress (ARDS) type syndrome. This may be due to aspiration, but it is possible that in patients with more severe neurogenic pulmonary oedema, the high permeability vascular damage may masquerade as ARDS.

The ECG at this stage (Figure 5.1) is surprising for a 32 year old previously fit woman with no history of ischaemic heart disease, and resembles an established anterior myocardial infarction. There are widespread Q wave changes, described in chapter 4, which have been shown to predict the subsequent development of neurogenic pulmonary oedema. It has also been mentioned that patients with sub-arachnoid haemorrhage have a tendency to arrhythmias. We have had experience of patients who have had sub-arachnoid haemorrhage occasionally going into ventricular fibrillation (VF) while having central lines or pulmonary artery (PA) catheters inserted. This happened in this patient, but defibrillation at 200 J restored normal rhythm and there were no further episodes of severe arrhythmia.

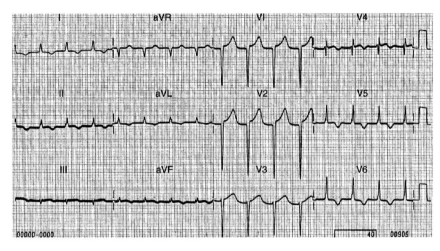

Figure 5.1   Electrocardiogram (ECG) tracing on day 2 showing T wave inversion and ST elevation.

Table 5.1   Effect of vasoactive therapy on day 2

	Initial value	After dobutamine, noradrenaline, and nimodipine
Heart rate (beats/min)	52	92
Mean arterial pressure (mmHg)	65	88
Pulmonary artery occlusion pressure (mmHg)	18	9
Cardiac index (L/min/m²)	2.4	5.8
Jugular oxygen saturation (%)	36	68
Intracranial pressure (mmHg)	20	20
Cerebral perfusion pressure (mmHg)	45	68
PaO_2 (kPa)	7.3	17.4
Fractional inspired oxygen	1	0.6

After insertion of a PA catheter the patient's ICP was 20 mmHg and her cerebral perfusion pressure was reduced at 45 mmHg. She was started on an infusion of dobutamine, noradrenaline (norepinephrine), and nimodipine. Table 5.1 shows the changes that occurred as a result of this therapy. Within a few hours, her heart rate and blood pressure were normal, she had a good cardiac output and much improved oxygenation. It is our experience that patients such as the case presented here do not tend to respond to nitrates, frusemide or CPAP in the way that patients with standard left ventricular failure often do.

41

Day 3

For the next 24 hours the patient remained sedated and as stated earlier she had developed neurogenic pulmonary oedema. In order to maintain her cerebral perfusion pressure noradrenaline was continued. Clearly adequate cardiac output and blood pressure are extremely important for the maintenance of cerebral perfusion pressure. It should be noted that administration of nimodipine should be done with care, because its vasodilatory action can catch you unawares. Even nasogastric nimodipine at a lower dose than that used intravenously can drop blood pressure and CPP. In the same way a loading dose of phenytoin given to convulsing patients can have such vasodilatory effects that all the previous haemodynamic achievements are lost.

Day 4

Over the subsequent 24 hours, our patient developed an elevated ICP and was treated with mannitol and frusemide. Osmolarity was measured routinely, as is our normal practice in patients receiving mannitol, and was increasing. The patient then developed sepsis in addition to the pulmonary complications already described. *Pneumococcus, Haemophilus influenzae* and *Staphylococcus aureus* were isolated from her tracheal secretions and she went on to develop septic shock.

Day 5

Over the next 24 hour period our patient was treated with noradrenaline 24 mg in 100 ml at a rate of 35 ml/hour. Her cardiac index was 9.9 L/min/m^2 and her mean arterial pressure was 83 mmHg. The nasogastric nimodipine dose was reduced to avoid haemodynamic problems. In addition, because of the increasingly high osmolarity and high ICP problems, a trial of hypnotic therapy (thiopentone) was attempted at

Table 5.2 Effect of dihydroergotamine on day 5

	Day 5 initial value	After dihydroergotamine
Mean arterial pressure (mmHg)	70	90
Intracranial pressure (mmHg)	30	30
Cerebral perfusion pressure (mmHg)	40	60
Jugular oxygen saturation (%)	78	70

this stage. However, this resulted in a fall in blood pressure and CPP, and, most worryingly, jugular venous oxygen saturation. Dihydroergotamine caused similar falls (Table 5.2) and this approach was therefore abandoned.

Days 5–12

The patient's ICP and CPP remained very unstable and she also became pyrexial. At this stage her ICP was 50 mmHg, CPP was 44 mmHg, jugular venous oxygen saturation was 77%, plasma sodium concentration was 160 mol/L, and osmolarity was 336 mosmol and rising. Hypnotic therapy was therefore re-attempted. She was given an etomidate bolus followed by a thiopentone infusion. The ICP decreased to 20 mmHg, CPP improved to 72 mmHg, and jugular bulb oxygen saturation was 60%. By day 12 the ICP gradually settled, the noradrenaline was gradually decreased, and the thiopentone was stopped. At this stage her GCS was 3.

On day 15 the patient was extubated and her GCS was 15. The following day she was discharged from the intensive care unit.

Her long-term outcome is excellent, with only mild weakness.

6: Sub-clinical seizures in the critically ill

ROGER E CULL

Introduction

The aim of this chapter is to provide a basic understanding of the types of seizures that may present on the intensive care unit (ICU). Neurophysiologists are quite often asked the question "Is this patient unconscious because they are having sub-clinical seizures?", and in my experience a positive answer is relatively unusual. Compared with other causes of unconsciousness in ICU patients, sub-clinical epileptic seizures are relatively uncommon.

Electroencephalography

Some of the electrical activity within the cerebral cortex can be detected using electrodes placed on the scalp, although this detects only a very small fraction of electrical activity in the brain. Using an array of electrodes provides some degree of spatial information. Several rhythmical waveforms identified by differing frequencies can be detected. With closed eyes, the most obvious frequency over the occipital cortex is 7–13/s and is known as the alpha rhythm. This disappears when the eyes are opened or sleep ensues. Other frequency bands seen over different parts of the brain in different circumstances are beta (faster than 13/s), theta (4–6/s), and delta (slower than 4/s). Lower frequencies predominate in the very young, and during sleep.

Evoked potentials

If a stimulus is provided–for example, to the eye – it would normally not be possible to detect the small response in electroencephalogram (EEG) that occurs over the occipital cortex, due to inherent background noise.

However, if data from several hundred repeated stimuli are electronically combined an averaged "evoked potential" can be detected. With appropriate positioning of electrodes, evoked potentials can be measured following either visual, auditory or somatosensory stimuli. Abnormalities of evoked potential indicate damage to the relevant pathway. The increased application of magnetic resonance imaging (MRI), has restricted the use of evoked potentials to certain specialised indications.

What is epilepsy?

A seizure can be defined as an abnormal clinical event caused by electrical discharge from the brain, and epilepsy is the tendency to have seizures. Epilepsy is a cerebral cortical phenomenon and represents a group of disorders. The seizures are characterised by altered cerebral function, which is associated with discharge of cortical neurones. Although the pathophysiology of epilepsy probably occurs through more than one mechanism, it is well recognised that during seizures there is excessive and hypersynchronous discharge of neurones and also probably some reciprocal inhibition either focally or generally in the cortex. In the normal cortex, synchronous discharge among neighbouring groups of neurones is limited by inhibitory discharges. The inhibitory neurotransmitter gamma-aminobutyric acid (GABA) is particularly important in this role and agents that block GABA receptors can provoke seizures. In epilepsy, cerebral cortex exhibits hypersynchronous repetitive discharges involving large groups of neurones. Intracellular recording show bursts of rapid-action potential firing, with reduction of the transmembrane potential (called paroxysmal depolarisation shift). Cells exhibiting these repetitive epileptic discharges undergo both morphological and physiological changes, which result in a susceptibility of the neurones to further abnormal discharges, a phenomenon known as kindling.

Classification of epilepsy

Since the early 1980s epilepsy has been further classified into two main groups: generalised seizures and partial seizures. Generalised seizures are those during which widespread paroxysmal activity is recordable on EEG. Partial seizures are those in which activity is more localised, although sometimes bilateral EEG changes are seen. Partial seizures are further classified into those that are simple, complex and partial with secondary generalisation. Generalised seizures are classified predominantly on the basis of their motor manifestations.

Partial seizures

Partial, or focal, seizures are those in which paroxysmal neuronal activity is limited to one part of the cerebrum, whereas in generalised seizures the electrophysiological abnormality involves both hemispheres of the brain simultaneously and synchronously. If partial seizures remain localised, the symptoms depend on the cortical area affected. If consciousness is preserved, the attack is termed "simple". If, however, the activity involves parts of the brain dealing with awareness (particularly the thalamus), then consciousness is affected and a "complex partial seizure" results. Further spread into the remainder of the cortex leads to a secondary generalised seizure.

Some partial seizures may be clinically inapparent (sub-clinical), or they may produce various clinical phenomena. Theoretically, the clinical manifestations of seizures are as diverse as cerebral function itself. In practice, seizures tend to occur in several recognisable patterns; therefore, a rational system of classification of seizures can be attempted (Box 6.1). Classifying seizures is useful because the cause, the likelihood of recurrence and the treatment of seizures vary depending on the type.

Box 6.1   Classification of seizures

Seizure type
- Simple partial
- Complex partial
- Absence
- Tonic–clonic
- Atonic
- Myoclonic

Anatomical site
- Cortex
  Temporal
  Frontal
  Parietal
  Occipital
- Generalised (diencephalon)
- Multifocal

Electrophysiology
- Focal waves/spikes
- Generalised spike and wave

Pathological cause

Simple partial seizures represent very focal activity, do not cause loss of awareness and do not always cause changes on the scalp EEG. Complex partial seizures cause some impairment of awareness, often total amnesia, and are associated with bilateral EEG paroxysmal activity. It is this type of seizure activity which usually causes impairment of consciousness and where other manifestations of epilepsy may not be apparent clinically.

Complex partial seizures are typically of temporal lobe origin but can arise from other cerebral areas such as the frontal, parietal or occipital lobes. The loss of awareness during the attacks is thought to imply some involvement of midline brain structures, especially the thalamus, by the epileptic discharge. Typical complex partial seizures last 1–3 minutes, but a prolonged state of partial seizure activity lasting hours can cause prolonged loss of awareness or confusion – called complex partial status epilepticus. Clinical clues to complex partial seizures are stereotyped automatism usually affecting the mouth (lip smacking, swallowing, belching) and upper limbs (semipurposeful finger movements, dystonic posturing), but these are not always present.

Generalised seizures

In primary generalised seizures, abnormal electrical activity begins synchronously throughout the cortex without an initial partial onset. It probably involves central diencephalic mechanisms interacting with cortical activation. This is seen as spikes and waves of abnormal activity on EEG (Figure 6.1). This may cause a major seizure or a more restricted clinical manifestation, such as loss of awareness if the abnormal electrical activity does not affect muscle tone. In this case there is loss of consciousness but the patient remains standing or sitting, and the attack may be difficult to distinguish clinically from a complex partial seizure in the temporal lobe. Generalised seizures can occur in primary generalised epilepsy, with an inherited tendency or as a result of spreading of complex partial seizure activity.

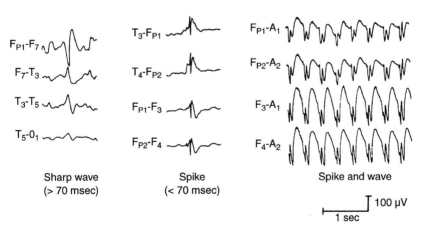

Figure 6.1   EEG tracings showing sharp waves, spikes and spike and wave epileptiform discharges. Reproduced from Westmoreland BF, Benarroch EE, Daube JR, Reagan TJ, Sandok BA. Medical neurosciences: an approach to anatomy, pathology, and physiology by systems and levels, 3rd edn. Boston: Little, Brown, 1994, pp. 249–271. By permission of Mayo Foundation.

Clinical manifestations of seizures

Generalised seizures

A tonic-clonic seizure may be preceded by a partial seizure, which can take various forms. However, the partial seizure often referred to as the "aura" may not be described due to subsequent seizure-related retrograde amnesia . The patient then goes rigid and loses consciousness. During this phase, respiration is arrested and evidence of cyanosis may be seen. After a few moments, the rigidity is periodically relaxed, producing clonic jerks. Some patients may not have a clonic phase and instead undergo a flaccid state of deep coma, which can persist for some minutes. The patient then gradually regains consciousness, but remains in a confused and disoriented state for some time after regaining consciousness. Full memory may not be recovered for some hours, and tiredness and headache occur. It should be noted that some patients may not have a characteristic tonic or clonic phase, and may not become cyanosed. However, post-seizure confusion and headache are usually seen. Psychogenic non-epileptic attacks, so called pseudo-seizures, may be accompanied by dramatic flailing of the limbs and arching of the back, but usually are not followed by the same degree of post-ictal confusion, and never cause cyanosis.

Generalised myoclonic seizures produce shock like body jerks, occurring singly or in succession, and are associated with generalised EEG discharges. Generalised tonic seizures cause sudden, sustained increased tone, most often manifested as flexor or extensor posturing. Air is often forced out of adducted vocal cords, and an unnatural and unmistakable guttural cry or grunt emanates. Generalised clonic seizures cause fairly symmetrical, bilateral, synchronous, semi-rhythmic jerking of the upper and lower extremities, usually with flexion at the elbows and extension at the knees. This jerking usually increases in amplitude and decreases in frequency as the seizure progresses and then ends after a few intermittent sporadic jerks. Generalised atonic seizures produce sudden, brief loss of tone that may cause abrupt falling; hence, they are often called "drop attacks". Many drop attacks are actually due to tonic seizures that affect the truncal musculature and propel the patient to the ground. Generalised seizures often evolve from tonic to clonic motor phenomena producing generalised tonic-clonic seizures. Brief myoclonic or clonic activity often precedes a more prolonged tonic-clonic seizure.

The EEG seen during generalised tonic-clonic seizure is literally a complete mixture with high frequency, high amplitude discharge and a certain amount of muscle activity. Immediately after the seizure high amplitude flows may be seen which may last for many minutes and up to an hour or two after the seizure. It is unlikely that major tonic-clonic seizures will be missed in patients on the ICU. However, when such patients are sedated and ventilated it is conceivable that it might not be apparent visually although such electrical activity will be seen even on two channel EEG. Changes in blood pressure and heart rate will also be apparent.

Complex partial seizures

Partial seizures may cause episodes of altered consciousness arising from the temporal or, less frequently, the frontal lobe. The patient stops what he or she is doing and stares blankly, often making rhythmic smacking movements of the lips or displaying other automatisms, such as picking at their clothes. After a few minutes the patient returns to consciousness but may be initially confused and drowsy. Immediately before such an attack the patient may report alterations of mood, memory and perception such as familiarity *déjà vu* or unreality *jamais vu*, complex hallucinations of sound, smell, taste, vision, emotional changes (fear, sexual arousal), or visceral sensations (nausea, epigastric discomfort). If these changes of memory or perception occur without subsequent alteration in awareness the seizure is a simple partial seizure.

Absence seizure

A type of minor seizure which resembles a complex partial seizure occurs in the generalised absence epilepsy of childhood, previously known as "petit mal". The attacks are usually briefer and occur more frequently (up to 30 per day in some cases) than complex partial seizures and are not associated with post-seizure confusion. Absence attacks are caused by a generalised discharge, which does not spread out of hemispheres and so does not cause loss of posture or consciousness.

Partial motor seizure

Epileptic activity arising in the precentral gyrus causes partial motor seizure affecting the contralateral face, arm, trunk, or leg. Such seizures are characterised by rhythmical jerking or sustained spasm of the affected parts and can vary in duration from a few seconds to several hours.

Conclusions

In summary, partial seizures are a relatively unusual cause of unconsciousness in ICU. The type of seizure most likely to contribute to the confusion is the complex partial seizure usually of temporal lobe origin; although typically a few minutes in duration, in some cases they can last longer. In most cases a routine 16 or 20 channel EEG will point to the diagnosis. However this may not be entirely specific because it may be dominated by rhythmical slow wave activity for which there are many causes, such as metabolic upset or drug intoxication.

Further reading

Cull RE, Will RG. Epilepsy. In: *Davidson's principles and practice of medicine*, 17th edn. Edinburgh: Churchill Livingstone, pp 1064–71.
Daube JR. *Clinical neurophysiology*. Philadelphia: FA Davis, 1996.
Mosewich RK, Elson L. A clinical approach to the classification of seizures and epileptic syndromes. *Mayo Clin Proc* 1996;**71**:405–14.
Westmoreland BF. Epileptiform electroencephalographic patterns. *Mayo Clin Proc* 1996;**71**:501–11.

7: Neurological injury in out-of-hospital cardiac arrest survivors: implications for management

NEIL R GRUBB, GRAHAM R NIMMO

Introduction

In the 1960s, pioneering emergency services initiatives paved the way for modern day out-of-hospital resuscitation programmes.[1-3] The introduction of a mobile coronary care unit (MCCU) in Belfast in 1966 led to the recognition that it is possible for individuals to survive ventricular fibrillation outside hospital.[1] Shortly after this, paramedic systems were introduced in Miami and in Seattle which demonstrated that cardiopulmonary resuscitation (CPR) and rapid defibrillation could be administered without the need for a doctor at the scene.[2,3] Subsequently, paramedic based out-of-hospital resuscitation programmes have been introduced in many major cities throughout the world.[4-8]

As a result of these initiatives, survival from out-of-hospital cardiac arrest is becoming an increasingly common occurrence. In the UK, survival rates from out-of-hospital cardiac arrest have increased in several cities.[9,10] Although prompt CPR and early defibrillation increase the probability of any given victim surviving their cardiac arrest, they also allow initial survival in people who would have otherwise succumbed immediately, only for them to die in hospital because of the sequelae of cerebral hypoxia. Thus, there is now an increasing population of cardiac arrest victims who survive with lethal or non-lethal brain injury. Of those who survive and are admitted to hospital, at least a third require management in an intensive care unit (ICU), mainly because of failure to spontaneously ventilate and self-oxygenate.[11] These resuscitated cardiac arrest victims present a challenge to intensivists in terms of assessing and managing neurological injury.

Information about co-morbidity is often not available when the patient arrives at the emergency room. Early neurological examination can be misleading because resuscitation drugs such as atropine and adrenaline (epinephrine) can interfere with pupillary responses. Yet this is the time when accurate and specific prediction of outcome would be most helpful in planning the most appropriate management for that individual. Accurate prognostic assessment of cardiac arrest survivors is an important task, because treatment decisions are often determined by these patients' prognoses. If the patient is considered to have no probability of survival to discharge, treatments such as CPR, antibiotic therapy or organ support may be deemed inappropriate. Equally, these patients should not be deprived of these treatments if their prospect of meaningful survival is real. In addition, knowledge about patients' prognoses helps when dealing with their families, especially when counselling about likely outcome.

Mechanisms of brain injury during and after cardiac arrest

Most of the existing information known about the mechanisms that lead to brain injury during and after cardiac arrest is derived from animal models, limited clinical studies of neonatal hypoxia, and studies of cerebral perfusion during cardiopulmonary bypass. These studies indicate that brain injury can occur through several mechanisms. Hypoxia itself is a major contributor, leading to failure of ATP-dependent cell membrane ion transporters, which in turn results in calcium influx into the cytoplasm, causing neuronal death. In addition, oxidative stress is now known to be a significant contributor to brain injury during the reperfusion phase.[12,13] At this time blood flow is abruptly restored, and oxygen is administered; the victim is suddenly subjected to supraphysiological oxygenation after a period of often prolonged, generalised hypoxia. Free radical-mediated tissue injury occurs, and can lead to microvascular damage and impaired reflow, similar to that seen after coronary reperfusion in myocardial infarction.[14,15] To compound this, cerebral oedema occurs early after reperfusion, because of movement of fluid from the intravascular compartment into the hyperosmotic interstitial space.[16] Infiltration of tissue by neutrophils may follow as a result of release of chemotactic factors and expression of integrins (eg, CD11b/CD18 and intercellular adhesion molecule 1 (ICAM-1)), and further tissue injury may result.[17] Finally, neuronal injury may also result from cerebral hypoperfusion in the post-resuscitation phase due to reduction in cardiac output. Collectively, these mechanisms form potential targets for interventions to potentially limit brain injury after cardiac arrest.

Prognostic assessment

Many different methods have been developed for assessing the prognosis of cardiac arrest victims. These include clinical algorithms, neurophysiological tests, and tests which quantify structural brain injury.

Clinical assessment

The ICU environment provides the best opportunity for neurological recovery of comatose cardiac arrest survivors. The key elements in this management are detailed below.

- Sedation and opioid analgesia.
- Mechanical ventilation via an endotracheal tube with the goal of optimising oxygenation and controlling $Paco_2$.
- Manipulation of the circulation with vasoactive drugs to maintain vital organ perfusion including cerebral perfusion pressure.

In this context it is difficult to fully assess motor and pupillary responses, but allowing sedative and analgesic drugs to wear off may not constitute optimum management for that patient.

Drugs and metabolic factors (Table 7.1) need to be considered as potential confounding factors when performing a clinical assessment.

Table 7.1   Confounding factors to clinical assessment

Drugs	Metabolic factors
Sedatives, eg benzodiazepines, opioids	Hypoxia and hypercarbia
Neuromuscular blockade	Temperature
Anticonvulsants	↑ or ↓ serum Na⁺
Antiarrhythmics, eg lignocaine	Cerebral perfusion pressure
	Hypoglycaemia

History

Broadly, the likelihood of hypoxic brain damage occurring is proportionate to the observed duration of cardiac arrest. However, estimating the duration of cardiac arrest is difficult, as the two most commonly cited time intervals are the estimated time from collapse to emergency call (from witness, and often inaccurate) and the time from the emergency call to successful defibrillation (often accurately assessed because defibrillator clocks are synchronised with those at the dispatch centre). However, the prognostic power of this may be reduced, because:

53

some patients may initially collapse with a low cardiac output state, and develop cardiac arrest later on; CPR is administered with variable frequency and competence; and cardiac arrests may be multiple, with further periods of cerebral hypoxia following the initial event.

Neurological examination

Several studies have examined the usefulness of neurological examination and clinical algorithms for prognostic assessment of patients with hypoxic coma. These studies have included patients with hypoxic coma due to shock and respiratory failure, as well as after cardiac arrest, and findings should be interpreted in the light of this. A sophisticated scoring system, incorporating variables such as pupil response, doll's eyes reflex, blink reflex, and presence or absence of seizures, was developed by Levy, based on data from more than two hundred patients with hypoxic-ischaemic coma.[18] From these data a flow-chart algorithm has been developed to predict prognosis at different time points after cardiac arrest. Age, sex and post-anoxic seizures were *not* predictive of outcome, a finding that has been reproduced in other studies. Interestingly, patients who had suffered cardiac arrest outside hospital achieved significantly better levels of independent outcome than those who had cardiac arrest in hospital. This type of algorithm is useful, and requires consistency in examination technique, but it is of limited use in patients receiving sedation or neuromuscular blockade.

In another study of 262 victims of cardiac arrest (both in- and out-of-hospital), absent pupil responses immediately on return of spontaneous circulation predicted poor neurological outcome in 88% of cases.[19] In both this and Levy's study, the presence of motor responses poorly predicted outcome within the first 48 hours of cardiac arrest, but after 72 hours, absent eye opening or pupil responses, or lack of motor response to pain, predicted poor outcome in all patients. These findings were recently substantiated in a systematic review by Zandbergen of 33 clinical and neurophysiological studies.[20]

Assessment of conscious level

Clinical assessment of conscious level aids risk stratification of cardiac arrest victims. The Glasgow Coma Score (GCS) is the most widely evaluated method.[21] Although a low GCS on admission identifies patients at high risk of death after admission to hospital, high specificity is only achieved when the GCS is measured three to five days after admission to hospital. Even at that point, patients with an intermediate GCS have an indeterminate prognosis, and use of the score is limited in sedated and ventilated patients. Verbal responses cannot be assessed after intubation, and motor and eye opening responses are affected by sedation and neuromuscular blockade. The Pittsburgh modified GCS adds little specificity, with both scales performing optimally when the patient is assessed at least 72 hours after the precipitating event.

Neurophysiological assessment

The two main techniques for neurophysiological assessment are electroencephalography (EEG), which measures cerebral electrical activity at rest, and somatosensory evoked potentials (SSEPs), which are measured in response to specific (eg, auditory) stimuli. Specific EEG findings, such as the alpha coma, burst suppression, and isoelectric patterns, are associated with an adverse prognosis.[20] However, these are not specific indicators and some patients survive despite their presence. By contrast, auditory evoked response potentials can reliably identify subgroups with a poor prognosis with superior specificity to clinical algorithms and the EEG. Zandbergen's review highlighted that bilateral absence of early cortical SSEPs in the first week after cardiac arrest had 100% specificity for predicting poor outcome.[20]

Quantification of brain injury

Clinical and neurophysiological techniques rely on assessing brain *function*. It is now also possible to estimate the magnitude of the brain *injury* caused by cardiac arrest. Magnetic resonance imaging and computerised tomography are not useful because they are poor at quantifying diffuse (as opposed to focal) injury. Usually only gross abnormalities such as watershed infarcts or intracranial haemorrhage can be seen. Brain injury can also be measured using biochemical markers, in the same manner as one uses measurement of cardiac enzymes to estimate the size of a myocardial infarction. Clinical studies indicate that two serum markers are useful – protein S-100 (a glial protein) and neuron-specific enolase (NSE). In one report a serum NSE concentration greater than 33 µg/l (any time within a week of cardiac arrest) had a sensitivity of 80% and a specificity of 100% for persistent coma.[22] Another report showed that measuring the serum S-100 concentration 24 hours after cardiac arrest identifies a subgroup with an apparently hopeless prognosis (S-100 concentration ≥0.7 µg/l).[23] These findings are not yet ready for clinical application because they are based on relatively small cohorts, and require confirmation in a larger scale study before these markers can be used to assist clinical decision making. At present, estimation of cerebral anoxic injury, as compared with brain function, has little use in the assessment of prognosis.

Clinical management

After admission, resuscitated cardiac arrest victims may be unstable for several reasons. Over a third are unable to adequately self-oxygenate, and require mechanical ventilation. Aspiration of gastric contents may exacerbate this problem. Peri-arrest arrhythmias are common, and guidelines for their management are published by the Resuscitation Council (UK).[24] Hypotension often occurs, both from the acute process that lead to the cardiac arrest (eg, myocardial infarction), and from post-resuscitation myocardial stunning. Peripheral vasomotor failure may result from hypoxia and hypoperfusion, and is mediated by release of cytokines and direct endothelial damage, compounding this tendency to hypotension. Inotropic agents and/or mechanical circulatory support are often needed to stabilise the patient in this early phase.

Reversible factors, such as electrolyte disturbance, pro-arrhythmic medication, systemic hypoxia, and sepsis should be sought during the initial assessment. If no obvious cause of cardiac arrest is found, a toxicology screen should be taken in case deliberate or accidental drug overdosage has occurred. Thereafter, other potential causes of cardiac arrest need to be identified.

Making appropriate decisions

It is worth noting that many resuscitated cardiac arrest victims are elderly and have serious underlying co-morbidity. An essential component of their management is involvement of family members in discussions about treatment. In this way, patients can be managed at a level appropriate to their overall prognosis and quality of life. However, age alone should not dictate whether or not intensive care is given, because the elderly have almost as good a prospect of survival to discharge as younger patients if they survive the cardiac arrest and reach hospital alive.[25]

Acute myocardial infarction – to treat or not?

Approximately 40% of out-of-hospital cardiac arrest victims have the underlying substrate of acute myocardial infarction.[9] Myocardial infarction is difficult to diagnose in cardiac arrest victims because the history may be absent or unclear, the ECG often shows an atypical pattern, and non-cardiospecific biochemical markers are deranged by trauma to skeletal muscle. Cardiospecific markers such as creatine kinase MB mass are extremely helpful in this situation.

The decision whether or not to give thrombolysis to these patients if they have received prolonged CPR is a difficult one. Trials do not provide consensus about the risk of serious haemorrhagic complications.[26-29] These complications include haemothorax and hepatic and retroperitoneal haemorrhage. The incidence of major bleeding has been reported to be as high as 19%, but most studies indicate that the risk is much lower than this. The approach has to be pragmatic – it seems reasonable to consider thrombolysis if there is a clear history of chest discomfort preceding collapse, conventional criteria for thrombolysis are met (Box 7.1), and there is no indication that the patient has suffered head trauma or a primary intracerebral haemorrhage. A CT head scan may be required to clarify this last issue. A chest X-ray should be checked before proceeding, because thrombolysis is contraindicated if significant thoracic trauma has occurred. As the benefits of thrombolysis are partly offset by the increased risk of haemorrhage in this group, it should probably be reserved for patients with a large infarct territory (eg, anterior infarction), or infarction with haemodynamic compromise.[29] If there is concern about the safety of thrombolysis, then primary angioplasty can be considered. Both primary angioplasty and thrombolysis salvage myocardium in most patients if they are given within eight hours of the onset of symptoms. Whether or not these are used, aspirin should be given either intravenously, or via a nasogastric tube. The only absolute contraindications are aspirin allergy and active gastrointestinal bleeding.

Box 7.1   Indications for thrombolysis

- Onset of typical ischaemic chest pain within previous 12 hours and

- ECG shows either:
  1 mm ST elevation in two or more adjacent limb leads or
  2 mm ST elevation in two or more adjacent chest leads or
  new left bundle branch block

Cardiac arrest without myocardial infarction

Most out-of-hospital cardiac arrest victims who have not had an acute myocardial infarction commonly have chronic ischaemic heart disease, often with a history of prior myocardial infarction and left ventricular impairment. In these patients, echocardiography helps identify structural substrates such as old infarct segments and left ventricular aneurysm. Other forms of structural or inherited heart disease that can cause cardiac arrest may also be identified, for example cardiomyopathies and valve defects. Detailed evaluation of the substrate of cardiac arrest is usually not performed until the patient's neurological prognosis is clear. At this point treatment options such as antiarrhythmic drugs and implantation of an automatic cardioverter-defibrillator (AICD) can be considered.

Intensive care management

Intensive care management, monitoring and support are often required after out-of-hospital cardiac arrest, for the reasons shown in Table 7.2.

Table 7.2   Reasons for intensive care admission

Indication	Management
Reduced conscious level	Airway maintenance, ventilation, neurological observation, CFAM
Oxygenation difficulties with:	
Cardiogenic shock	IPPV, high Fio$_2$, PEEP
Left ventricular failure	IPPV, high Fio$_2$, PEEP
Aspiration / ARDS	IPPV, high Fio$_2$, PEEP, IRV, NO, prone positioning
Haemodynamic instability:	
Low cardiac output	Inotropes, IABP
Peripheral vasomotor failure	Vasopressors, IABP
Arrhythmias	Drugs, pacing, IABP, etc.
Seizures	Anticonvulsants, anaesthesia, CFAM

CFAM = cerebral function analyser and monitor, Fio$_2$ = fractional inspired oxygen, IABP = intra-aortic balloon pump, IPPV = intermittent positive pressure ventilation, IRV = inverse ratio ventilation, NO = nitric oxide, PEEP = positive end expiratory pressure ventilation.

Sedation and paralysis

The combination of alfentanil and propofol infusions is useful for these patients, because the rapid offset allows neurological assessment comparatively soon after withdrawal. However, in patients with haemodynamic instability, short-acting benzodiazepines such as midazolam may be better tolerated. Neuromuscular paralysis, in many cases, is not required and is best avoided if possible. If it is used, continuous monitoring of cerebral electrical activity (eg, cerebral function analyser and monitor, CFAM) should be carried out to allow detection and treatment of seizure activity. Indications for neuromuscular blockade include precarious oxygenation despite high Fio$_2$ (eg, requiring inverse ratio ventilation), or very low cardiac output and oxygen delivery (to limit oxygen consumption).

Intermittent positive pressure ventilation

Standard IPPV with tidal volumes of 10–12 ml/kg is often sufficient if there are no problems with pulmonary compliance. Inverse ratio (IRV) or pressure control ventilation may become necessary if oxygenation is problematical using this regime. If IRV or high pressure positive end expiratory pressure (PEEP) are used, cardiac output may be compromised, and should be monitored and supported with inotropes if necessary. Ideally ventilation should aim to achieve a target PaO_2 greater than 11 kPa, and $PaCO_2$ between 4 and 4.5 kPa.

Seizures

Seizures can be controlled with standard measures, using benzodiazepines for acute treatment and phenytoin to prevent recurrence. The loading dose of intravenous phenytoin is 10–15 mg/kg, but can cause significant hypotension at this dose. Dividing the dose into two, administered several hours apart, minimises this effect. In status epilepticus, propofol or thiopentone can be used to abolish seizure activity if these measures fail.

Haemodynamic management

An arterial line and central venous catheter are normally used to aid haemodynamic monitoring. Hypotension, as mentioned earlier, may arise due to low cardiac output, impaired vasoconstriction, arrhythmias, or a combination of these factors. If hypotension occurs, early echocardiography provides useful information about left ventricular function. Pulmonary artery catheterisation is often needed in the complex patients with low cardiac output, as this allows assessment of cardiac output and pulmonary artery wedge pressure. Inotropic support and pressor treatment are guided by these indices, and are used to maintain blood pressure (and hence cerebral and coronary perfusion pressure). Monitoring of mixed venous oxygen saturation gives prognostically important information, and assists titration of inotropes, to minimise the attendant risks of myocardial ischaemia and arrhythmias.[30] To maintain systemic oxygen delivery and the myocardial oxygen supply/demand balance, oxygen carrying capacity may need to be optimised with red cell transfusion to a haemoglobin concentration of 120 g/l or greater.

General management

Maintenance of strict metabolic control may aid recovery of cerebral function. Avoidance of secondary cerebral insults is known to benefit patients with traumatic brain injury, and a similar approach is likely to help comatose cardiac arrest survivors. Hypotension and systemic hypoxia should be treated as detailed above. Hypoglycaemia, hyperglycaemia and hyponatraemia should be avoided, with scrupulous attention to fluid management, avoiding dextrose infusions. Pyrexia should be treated using cooling measures and paracetamol. Chest infection is common, particularly with *Haemophilus influenzae*, *Streptococcus pneumoniae* and *Staphylococcus aureus*. If aspiration has occurred, anaerobic infection may also contribute. If purulent secretions are evident, broad spectrum intravenous antibiotic therapy should be initiated (including anaerobic cover, eg, metronidazole) after blood and sputum samples have been obtained for culture. A nasogastric tube should be sited, to allow enteral feeding.

Future directions – neuroprotection?

Many treatments attempting to limit cerebral damage after cardiac arrest have been assessed. These include administration of glucose (as a substrate for brain metabolism), dexamethasone and mannitol (to reduce osmotic load and cerebral oedema), barbiturates (to reduce cerebral oxygen demand), and nimodipine (to improve cerebral blood flow and to reduce entry of calcium into neurones). None of these agents have been shown conclusively to improve outcome. An encouraging development in neuroprotection is signalled by experimental evidence of limitation of brain injury using antioxidant agents, notably the 21-aminosteroid tirilazad.[31] Because oxidative stress may cause additional brain injury several hours after cardiac arrest, antioxidants may have a future role in neuroprotection.

Long-term outcomes – quality of survival

Cardiac arrest victims who survive the early phase may have suffered a damaging episode of cerebral hypoxia. The resulting neurological injury can be severe enough to affect cognitive function, and to compromise patients' independence. Surprisingly, overt neurological deficits are relatively uncommon, affecting less than 5% of patients. Cognitive dysfunction is more prevalent, affecting between 20% and 50% of patients.[14] Memory impairment is common and may affect the patient's ability to return to work and to perform daily activities. Despite this, most out-of-hospital cardiac arrest survivors are functionally independent and have intact cognitive function.

Conclusions

Management of comatose out-of-hospital cardiac arrest victims is not an easy task. The key elements of initial management are early assessment of ventilatory status, identification of underlying myocardial infarction, and optimisation of haemodynamic, cerebral and ventilatory function in the intensive care unit. The degree to which interventions are employed needs to take account of patients' quality of life, co-morbidity and prognosis. Thus, early communication with patients' relatives is important, and use of prognostic assessments, such as clinical scoring systems and neurophysiological parameters, both contribute to the management of these patients. Although more than half die despite our best efforts, those patients who survive usually do so with a relatively good quality of life.

References

1 Pantridge JF, Geddes JS. A mobile intensive care unit in the management of myocardial infarction. *Lancet* 1967;**ii:**271–3.

2 Liberthson RR, Nagel EL, Hirschmann JC, Nussenfeld SR. Prehospital ventricular defibrillation: prognosis and follow-up course. *N Engl J Med* 1974;**291:**317–21.

3 Cobb LA, Werner JA, Trobaugh GB. Sudden cardiac death: I. A decade's experience with out-of-hospital resuscitation. *Mod Concepts Cardiovasc Dis* 1980:**49:**31–6.

4 Muisma M, Määttä T. Out-of-hospital cardiac arrests in Helsinki: Utstein style reporting. *Heart* 1996;**76:**18–23.

5 Weaver WD, Cobb LA, Hallstrom AP, Fahrenbruch C, Copass MK, Ray R. Factors influencing survival after out-of-hospital cardiac arrest. *J Am Coll Cardiol* 1986;**7:**752–7.

6 de Vreede-Swagemakers JJ, Gorgels APM, Dubois-Arbuow WI, van Ree JW, Daeman M, Houben LG, Wellens HJ. Out-of-hospital cardiac arrest in the 1990s: a population-based study in the Maastricht area on incidence, characteristics and survival. *J Am Coll Cardiol* 1997;**30:**1500–5.

7 White RD, Asplin BR, Bugliosi TF, Hankins DG. High discharge survival rate after out-of-hospital ventricular fibrillation with rapid defibrillation by police and paramedics. *Ann Emerg Med* 1996;**28:**480–5.

8 Gaul GB, Gruska M, Titscher G, *et al.* Prediction of survival after out-of-hospital cardiac arrest: results of a community-based study in Vienna. *Resuscitation* 1996;**32:**169–76.

9 Cobbe SM, Redmond MJ, Watson JM, Hollingworth J, Carrington DJ. "Heartstart Scotland" – initial experience of a national scheme for out of hospital defibrillation. *Br Med J* 1991;**302:**1517–20.

10 Dickey W, McKenzie G, Adgey AAJ. Long-term survival after resuscitation from ventricular fibrillation occurring before hospital admission. *Q J Med* 1991;**80:**729–37.

11 Grubb NR, Elton R, Fox KAA. In-hospital mortality after out-of-hospital cardiac arrest. *Lancet* 1995;**346:**417–21.

12 Callaway CW, Kagan VE, Kochanek PM. Electron spin resonance

measurement of brain antioxidant activity during ischemia/reperfusion. *Neuroreport* 1998;**9**:1587–93

13 Palmer C. Hypoxic-ischaemic encephalopathy, therapeutic approaches against microvascular injury, and role of neutrophils, PAF and free radicals. *Clin Perinatol* 195;**22**:481–517.

14 White BC, Gross LI, O'Neill BJ, *et al.* Global brain injury and reperfusion. *Ann Emerg Med* 1996;**27**:588–94.

15 Bottiger BW, Krumniki JJ, Gass P, Schmitz B, Motsch J, Martin E. The cerebral "no-reflow" phenomenon after cardiac arrest in rats – influence of low flow reperfusion. *Resuscitation* 1997;**34**:79–87.

16 Jannucci RC, Christensen MA, Yagen JY. Nature, time course and extent of cerebral edema in perinatal hypoxic-ischemic brain damage. *Paediatr Neurol* 1993;**9**:29–34.

17 Howard EF, Chen Q, Cheng C, Carroll JE, Hess D. NF-kappa B is activated and ICAM-1 gene expression is upregulated during reoxygenation of human brain endothelial cells. *Neurosci Lett* 1998;**248**:199–203.

18 Levy DE, Caronna JJ, Singer BH, Lapinski RH, Frydman H, Plum F. Predicting outcome from hypoxic-ischaemic coma. *JAMA* 1985;**253**:1420–6.

19 Edgren E, Hedstrand U, Kelsey S, Sutton-Tyrrell K, Safar P and BRCT 1 study group. Assessment of neurological prognosis in comatose survivors of cardiac arrest. *Lancet* 1994;**343**:1055–9.

20 Zandbergen EGJ, de Haan RJ, Stoutenbeek CP, Koelman JHTM, Hijdra A. Systematic review of early prediction of poor outcome in anoxic-ischaemic coma. *Lancet* 1998;**352**:1808–12.

21 Verbruggen H, Van den Brock L, Corne L, Lauwaert D. Predictive value of Glasgow coma score for awakening after out-of-hospital cardiac arrest. Cerebral Resuscitation Study Group of the Belgian Society for Intensive Care. *Lancet* 1988; **i**(8578):137–40.

22 Barone FC, Clark RK, Price WJ, *et al.* Neuron-specific enolase increases in cerebral and systemic circulation following focal ischaemia. *Brain Research* 1993;**623**:77–82.

23 Martens P, Raabe A, Johnsson P. Serum S-100 and neuron specific enolase for prediction of regaining consciousness after global cerebral ischaemia. *Stroke* 1998;**29**:2363–6.

24 Chamberlain D. Peri-arrest arrhythmias. *Br J Anaesth* 1997;**79**:198–202.

25 Juchems R, Wahlig G, Frese W. Influence of age on the survival rate of out-of-hospital and in-hospital resuscitation. *Resuscitation* 1993;**26**:23–9.

26 Druwe PM, Cools J, De Raedt HJ, Bossaert LL. Liver rupture after cardiopulmonary resuscitation in a patient receiving thrombolytic therapy. *Resuscitation* 1996;**32**:213–16.

27 Tenaglia AN, Califf RM, Candela RJ, *et al.* Thrombolytic therapy in patients requiring cardiopulmonary resuscitation. *Am J Cardiol* 1991;**68**:1015–19.

28 Scholz KH, Tebbe U, Herrmann C, *et al.* Frequency of complications of cardiopulmonary resuscitation after thrombolysis during acute myocardial infarction. *Am J Cardiol* 1992;**69**:724–8.

29 The ISIS-2 Collaborative Group. Randomized trial of intravenous streptokinase, oral aspirin, both or neither among 17 817 cases of suspected acute myocardial infarction: ISIS-2. *Lancet* 1988;**ii**:349–60.

30 Nimmo GR, Grant IS, Mackenzie SJ. Lactate and acid base changes in the critically ill. *Postgrad Med J* 1991;**67**(suppl 1):S56–61.

31 Sterz F, Janata K, Kurciyan I, Mullner M, Malzer R, Schreiber W. Possibilities of brain protection with tirilazad after cardiac arrest. *Semin Thromb Haemostasis* 1996;**22**:105–12.